MIRACLE IN RICHARDS BAY

Escape From The Vortex

By

Maya Knight

'Miracle in Richards Bay - Escape from the Vortex' by Maya Knight

Copyright © 2021 - Maya Knight.
First printing 2021
Design and layout - Maya Knight and Sweetfields Publishing
956 Comboyne Rd, Cedar Party, NSW Australia 2429
Edited by Anna Rose
cover by Maya and Trevor Knight
P.O. Box 179, Bulahdelah, N.S.W. Australia 2423

email:- maya.palmist@gmail.com
Internet:- www.mayaknight.com.au

ISBN:- 978-0-6485538-1-6

A catalogue record for this book is available from
The National Library of Australia, Canberra, ACT, Australia

Set in Times New Roman font.

Reproduction in any manner, in whole or in part, in
English or in any other language, or otherwise,
without the written permission of the copyright
holder is prohibited

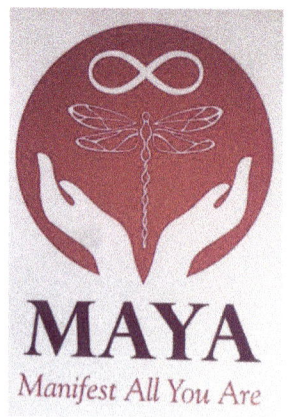

DEDICATION

I would like to dedicate this book to my wonderful husband, Trevor. He showed me the meaning of unconditional love.

When we made our wedding vows I know we both did so believing that we would stick by each other in sickness and in health and for better or worse but we often don't know the reality of what that might really entail – I do now!

It's not till we are truly tested that we can really know ourselves, and although this was not something we chose to go through, we did so together with our love and respect guiding and supporting us.

Trevor, you were my strength when I needed it most, my hope when I lost sight of it and throughout everything, you were my friend, my confidant …my everything. Thank you.

I also want to thank my wonderful family (Kristy, Hans, Rowena, Steven, Mark, Jaydn, Matthew, Jake, Liam, Bronwyn, Tony, Tristan, Rene, Penelope, Anghus, Theodore, Brian, Jenny, Robert, Chas, Rene and Delma) for your unwavering support, love and prayers.

Next, let me say a special thank you to my friends in Australia (you know who you are and how much I appreciated your love and best wishes).

Also a big 'thank you' to my 'new' amazing friends who took time almost every day to visit me and brighten my days. (Sharmilla, Angelique, Tamsin, Pastor Cecil Pillay and his family and congregation and all those wonderful people we interacted with each and every day who touched our lives including Kenneth, Michael and Gabriel.

Next, words fail me in my thanks to Doctor Kritish Timakia as well as Doctor Lucelle Padayachee and the team in Intensive Care. You saved my life . . . literally. I certainly would not have been here to 'tell the tale' without YOU. You are all angels in my eyes.

And last but no means least, Trevor and I owe a big debt to Princess Cruises who came to our aid and were always there supporting us in so many ways.

Maya

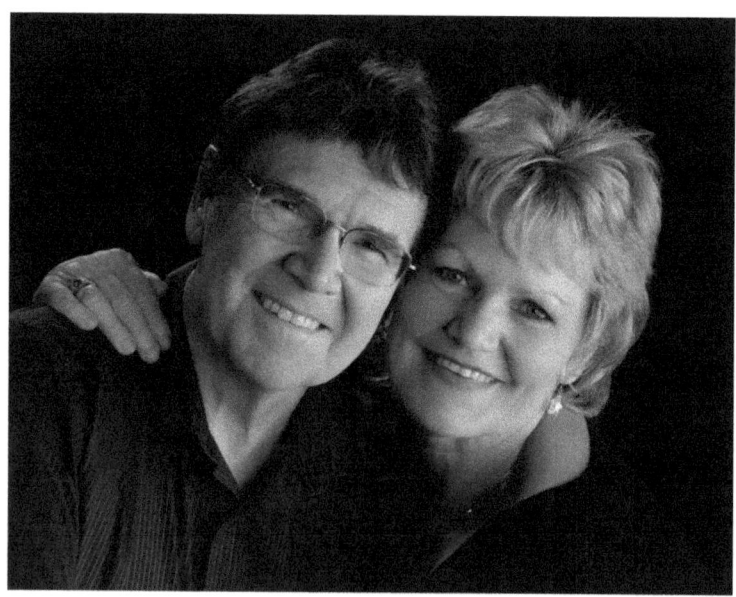

Dr. Timakia's Foreward

The year 2020 was the start of a difficult era for society as at no other time have we had to bear the burden of being isolated from our friends and family, in the hope that it would be beneficial to these very individuals.

The experience of being isolated, alone and facing a probable life-threatening situation in 2020, is an unfathomable one.

This was the surreal reality Maya [sharing my wife's name], faced when she walked onto South African soil.

The course of events, her recovery and efforts to return home across the planet, all within a month, can only be appreciated now in hindsight.

The sequences of events in the lives of all those involved in her care and return home all led us from that moment when we met.

Whether it was divine intervention or just part of our Universe's plan, I am grateful that I had the opportunity to meet with both Maya and Trevor and be a part of their lives.

Their request was the simplest request a person could make - they needed help and I was so glad I could help make this happen for them, as I would for anyone coming to me.

So in hindsight, I wonder how I could not appreciate the gravity of this experience.

Maya and Trevor walked onto South African soil where she was diagnosed with a life-threatening brain tumour that needed urgent medical intervention and treatment and rehabilitation.

Whilst there, they met and made life-long friends (including me) and then flew back to Australia in the nick of time before being totally locked out for months due to this pandemic spreading the globe.

Our lives are shaped by the experiences we have and the people we meet along our path and I am truly grateful to have met Maya and Trevor.

Since their departure, I have kept in contact to let them know about the birth of my son and it was wonderful that they shared my happiness in this moment.

I hope that this experience is an example and reminder to people that prayers are answered and to always hold firm our faith in the kindness of humanity.

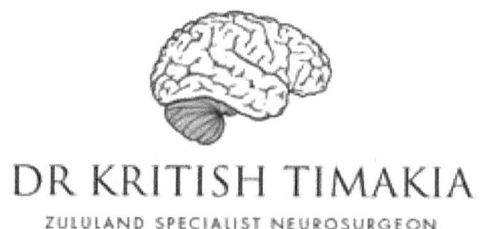

DR KRITISH TIMAKIA

ZULULAND SPECIALIST NEUROSURGEON

EDITOR'S NOTE

It was my absolute pleasure to edit Maya's magnificent book. What a page-turner!

You have in your hands one of the most thrilling and heart-warming human-interest stories I've come across in more than 30 years of journalism.

The fact that Maya and Trevor found each other in the first place gladdened my heart. Not everyone finds their one true love. Throughout the book you will get to know the depth of their love and their deep respect for each other.

The incredible support they both received from their respective families and from their newfound friends in Zululand is to be admired.

To face what they both did, knowing that their lives could change in the flicker of an eye, then to come out the other end smiling, truly was a miracle.

My advice to you is to make a warm drink (or a cool one), find a cosy spot to sit and prepare to lose yourself for a day or so. This is one book you'll never forget.

Anna Rose
Journalist/editor/sub-editor and author
August 2021

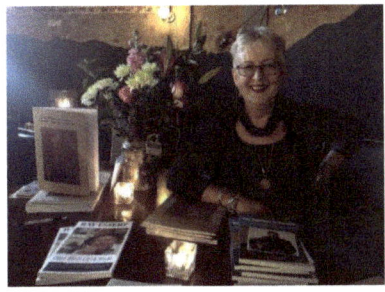

'Miracle in Richards Bay - Escape from the Vortex' by Maya Knight

Coincidence is God's way Of remaining anonymous

Einstein

Birth... Death
And everything in between is life;
Your Life.

Some people count the minutes, the hours,
the days the years.

Others laugh, dance, sing and love.
They make every moment count.

Which one are you?
With every choice; with every decision,
You choose the life you want to live.

CHAPTER 1

It's noon and I'm waiting patiently just outside the theatre ... only this is far from the theatre I had hoped to be performing in, and I'm not the one on centre stage.

Instead, I'm in my hospital bed in the intensive care unit (ICU) at the Netcare Bay Hospital in Richards Bay, South Africa, 10,500 miles from home. I have lost most of my ability to verbally communicate. My right side is getting weaker every day and my mouth is markedly lower on the right side.

I feel so strange in this body that is letting me down on so many levels. It's like I am in two minds ... one that just doesn't respond any more to what I want to express or say, and the other one that fully comprehends and understands everything that's going on.

I'm glad in some ways that I have to wait a little longer because it gives me a bit more time with Trevor, my wonderful husband ... it might be the last time I will ever see him, and I want to treasure every single minute we have together.

Funny how time can become so precious; and it reminds me of all those moments that I took for granted.

But that's what happens in life. We have so much to be grateful for, that it often becomes ho-hum and we forget what's important ... until there is a very real threat to it, or the possibility we may lose it forever.

In fact, that's exactly what I say in my lectures about *Success and Happiness in the Palm of your Hand*.

As I was being wheeled to the operating theatre, I was reminded of this and I questioned myself ...

Did I live an authentic life ... a life as me?

Did I utilise every gift that was given to me?

Did I live my life to the fullest?

Did I really get the best out of me and give the best of me?

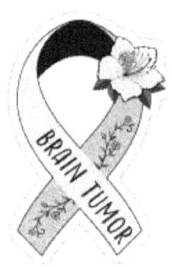

*Greatness is nothing short of
'Wholeness of purpose'*

Trust in the truth that comes with a life lived true and full.

*Always do your very best
Always strive
Always be true and go forward.*

CHAPTER 2

I had been a regular inspirational speaker and authority on palmistry on cruise ships and I always encouraged people to really value 'who' they are. I always believed that to be the full expression of 'you' is your path to happiness and fulfillment.

When I did these talks, little did I realise that one day, I would be the one who couldn't express myself.

It wasn't that I didn't want to. It was because I was no longer able to, and in that moment, I realised that our ability to communicate is probably one of our greatest gifts, certainly one of mine.

I was learning the real value of communicating firsthand, because not only had I lost it; I might never get it back again.

As I did this mini appraisal on my life, I realised I'd dedicated my life to areas that were so dependent upon communication. I had worked in mental health as a registered psychiatric nurse for more than forty years (the majority of my life) and I was also an internationally renowned psychic palmist.

In my job as a nurse, I was no stranger to the tragedies of life … the young man whose future is shattered by the diagnosis of schizophrenia; the mother who murdered her baby because she believed she had to kill the evil in her child and present her to God; the many women, and often men, who abuse themselves over and over because as children they were abused again and again in the worst possible ways; the lost, empty, depressed souls who believe their only option is suicide, and so many lives ruined directly or indirectly by the impact of mental illness. It affects them, not only in their relationships, but also in their abilities to function in this world.

It's funny how I fell into this role because it was so far from my childhood dreams. I always wanted to become a home economics teacher. I just loved to cook and sew, and I still do. However, after I left high school at age seventeen, I didn't want to go straight into teachers' college ... I wanted a bit of a break.

I ended up doing odd jobs to bring in some money, but I really couldn't settle into anything. Then I saw an advertisement for psychiatric nursing assistants and thought: 'That might be good for a few months' – after all, the money was good.

I was so naïve in those days and really had no idea about mental illness and the tragedies surrounding people afflicted by it, or the impact on their friends and families.

It's so amazing as we look back upon the tapestry we weave throughout our lives, and the turns and crossroads that lead us to a destiny we are often not even aware is our true calling. Looking back over my life, I came to see that everything in my personality and all the skills I honed over the years that made me so approachable, empathetic, sensitive and intuitive were there right from the start and all I had to do was hone and polish them.

Over the years I've certainly cried many times for the tragedy that is severe mental illness, but I've also laughed. It's how humans work. It's nature's release valve for the psyche and I've always been very conscious of keeping my own mental health in check by living a well-balanced, creative, happy life to compensate for the times of pressure and stress this job inflicts.

It quite surprised me that not only did I stay in this job, I also went on to do my training to become a fully qualified psychiatric nurse.

Imagine my amazement as well when I came second in the final state examination. I remember the other class members all swatting up beforehand and I kept thinking I was going to fail because I just didn't seem to have the same slant on things as they did. This was perhaps my first big lesson in life about being true to me and not second guessing myself.

However, old habits die hard, and over the years, despite what I told others, I had continued to have an issue with comparing myself with others and believing that I fell short.

My first day on the job was such an eye-opener. I was working a morning shift and was assigned to work 'on the hill'. I reported to the nurse-in-charge who told me my job was to clean the bathrooms before, during and after the 30 or so bedridden children and young intellectually challenged and autistic children and young adults were woken up, showered, fed and put back in their cots.

I was overwhelmed by the stench of the place. Some of the children were lying in their own excrement and had foul-smelling breath because no-one seemed to have time to do proper oral hygiene. If the walls could have talked, they would have spoken of the misery that was the lives of these poor souls.

I was appalled by the lack of hygiene as well as the lack of interpersonal interactions staff had with the patients. However, the thing that appalled me even more, was the expectation placed upon a team of four nurses.

Together, we had to do everything for these children and young adults. This included cleaning, bathing, feeding them and giving them tablets as well as cleaning the ward. Each ward housed from 30 to 40 patients. The standards were very poor, and to this day, I wondered why I stayed. It was heartbreaking to see the lack of love and care, and to know that most of these children had been dumped and disowned by their own families.

The food they were given was colloquially referred to as 'Woogaroo stew'. It was minced meat and vegetables in a thick gravy. They were given this morning, noon and night. There were no treats. There was no one to sing to them or give them cuddles or to make them feel loved. Many of them had no visitors and certainly nothing to look forward to in life.

Although I wanted to do more, I was unable to, because it was a really strict system I worked under and there was a definite chain of command, with me being very low on the rung.

Thank God, due to a big revision in the administration of nursing care, these wards were closed down soon after I started working there.

I was never the ambitious type, aspiring for power and position, but I very much wanted to see changes happen and be able to be instrumental in this process. I wanted to make a difference in people's lives, so they felt they were valued and had the right to dream and have a real say in their own lives.

Realising there was only one way I could do this, I began to apply for higher positions. As a registered nurse, I certainly had some input, but the system was such that there were many bullies who would override these, and I didn't have a leg to stand on in the environment that prevailed at that time (this was the '70s and '80s when psychiatric care in Queensland was still very much in the dark ages).

It was interesting because at this time my brother Hans was living in Sydney, and despite having done his psychiatric nursing training several years before I did at Wolston Park Hospital (where I was based), he was made to redo it all as they did not recognise the training he'd already had.

He recalls being shown a film, *The Seven Ages of Psychiatry*. This showed nursing care supposedly '50 years ago' and he told me this was the way he'd remembered it in Queensland, only it hadn't been 50 years ago – it had been less than five years ago.

By the time I was doing my training in the late 1970s, there were quite a few improvements being implemented, but also a lot of resistance to the way things used to be. A lot of the 'old' staff preferred working in the chronic wards whereas the newer staff and students were allocated to work in the more acute areas. There was also this wonderful 'radically new' idea of working with patients (as we called them then) in the community. This was something that was already implemented in New South Wales and Victoria and we copied their model of care.

In 1988 I became a clinical nurse consultant and concurrently, I did a course at Griffith University where I got my Graduate Diploma in Community Mental Health Nursing – again achieving very high marks.

This led to some of the most fulfilling times in my nursing career. Together with a small team of nurses, psychologists, psychiatrists and social workers, we set up a community integrated mental health service in the West Moreton Area of South-East Queensland.

I worked in both the assessment team, where we largely visited people in their homes to do face-to-face assessments, as well as telephone assessments. I also worked in the mobile intensive treatment team, which did exactly what it sounds like it did.

This was certainly not a team for the faint-hearted. We had almost daily contact with our clients doing whatever was needed to keep them safe, well, and in the community. We learned to build very strong, therapeutic relationships with our clients, and this is really where I learned the true hardships these people face, the least of them being discrimination.

Through consistent interactions in all sorts of environments, I got to understand the fears that came up for a lot of my clients. Loneliness and financial constraints were huge issues. Added to this were the thought processes, often delusional and totally irrational, that would drive some of their behaviours. A lot of them had trust issues and issues with getting into healthy relationships, let alone maintaining them. Sadly, most had been ostracised by family and friends as well so had very little, if any social life or social supports.

This understanding led me to learning about true compassion and acceptance of people as they are. I became very focused on looking at the possibilities within people and also around them, and helping them to not only see these, but to manifest them in their lives. This is often the most difficult thing to do because it's a matter of pushing through people's own limiting self-beliefs, as well as the limiting beliefs imposed upon them by others in the past and in the present.

We continued our support with our clients if they needed admission to the in-patient unit and we were a big part of their discharge planning, so admissions became not only less frequent, but also not as long.

I became fascinated with what makes people think the way they do and although I wasn't really interested in the biology of how the brain works, I was fascinated and wanted to get a deeper understanding of thoughts and why people think the sort of thoughts they do.

I especially loved the idea that we can train our brains to work in our favour by feeding it properly with positive input as well as great nutrition. Most of my personal philosophies are based around this.

One of my favourite sayings is:

> Changing my thinking
> Changes my beliefs,
> Which changes my expectations,
> Which then changes my attitude,
> Which changes my behaviour,
> Which changes my performance,
> Which changes my life.

'Miracle in Richards Bay - Escape from the Vortex' by Maya Knight

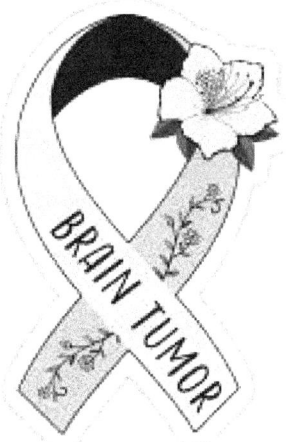

You must clear the barriers
In order to fulfill your purpose
And shine a light
For others to follow.

Then and only then
Will you be on your path.

Reach to the hands
That pull you up,
Not to the thumbs
That hold you down.

CHAPTER 3

I was born in The Netherlands on July 3, 1956. This was a good time in lots of ways. The war had been over for a number of years and people had started to rebuild their lives, with some, including my parents, becoming quite prosperous.

My dad was an engineer and had worked on ships up until the time he got married at age 28. He used to reminisce frequently about this romantic time in his life – a life of sailing and adventure. This was his 'safe topic' and although he was very clever and could turn his hands to nearly anything, he had problems discussing his feelings and could never admit to being wrong. Saying sorry was impossible for him.

He was a very proud man and the transition from the life as a sailor to a husband and father was a difficult one.

On the other hand, my mother was very family orientated, being one of eleven children. Her parents would also foster children from time to time. Her family kept in very close contact, and although not openly loving, they were very close to each other and showed this throughout their lives with constant contact by mail and later, phone calls.

In 1957, my father broached the idea of immigrating to Australia. My mum was not too keen initially, but with three children and the horrors of war behind her, plus the fear of another war, she wanted to feel safe herself and wanted a place that could offer her children a better life.

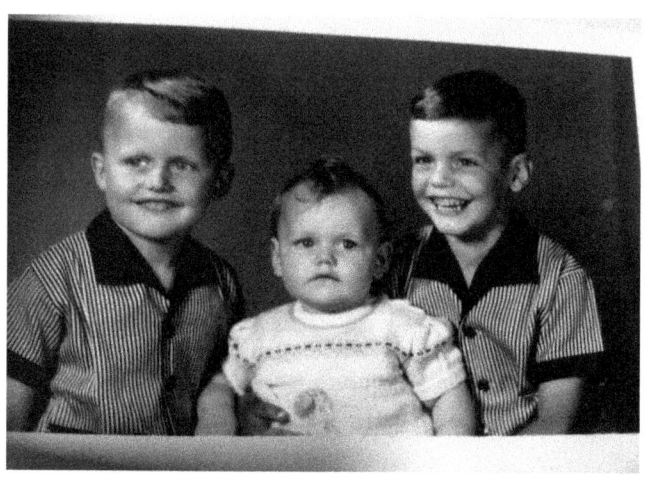

Hans, Sylvo and me, as a one year old.

Her elder brother had moved to Australia several years before this and had said he would help them get settled. However, after selling up most of their beautiful furniture and belongings and expecting him to be there waiting for them, they were most disappointed to learn he wasn't really able to help or support them, nor did he have the contacts he had indicated he did.

As a result, our family spent four years in a migration camp in Wacol (one of the western suburbs of Brisbane, Queensland). This was a difficult time for them (to say the least). The five of us (and in 1959 after the birth of my sister, Ingrid, the six of us) lived in a tiny army hut.

Although my father got a job quite soon after we arrived in Australia, it was as a fitter and turner (a little beneath his qualifications). Like many migrants, despite what he had been led to believe, Australia would not recognise his previous qualifications.

Their only mode of transport was bicycle and although bikes were great in Holland where the country is beautifully flat, here in Australia, riding a bicycle can be a bit challenging (especially one without gears). This is how my father completed the daily 10km-plus trip to and from work, come rain, shine, heat or cold.

Then disaster struck.

About 1959, two years after we migrated to Australia, my father was diagnosed with a rare illness, Buerger's disease (thromboangiitis obliterans). This disease causes the small blood vessels, particularly in the extremities, to become inflamed, resulting in reduced blood flow, ultimately causing them to become gangrenous. The disease is largely related to younger men who smoke tobacco.

As the disease progressed, he would experience many months of excruciating pain, with the hope that his fingers and toes could be saved. Unfortunately, this was rarely the case, and would require surgical intervention.

Over the years he had to have five toes surgically removed as well as five segments of his fingers.

He had to be extremely careful at work because any injury, no matter how minor, could trigger the disease and months off work would follow. This led to depression (though he could never admit to this) and lots of emotional problems, as he tried to come to terms with the many issues and losses he had to deal with in an unfamiliar environment.

I remember many times, seeing him rocking as he sat outside on the verandah, moaning in pain. It was dreadful to witness because he was such a tough man.

My father worked at the Morris Woollen Mills doing the afternoon shift, which meant we saw very little of him. He was such a respected and valuable worker, that despite all the months he needed to have off work due to the impact of his disease, his job was always there for him.

Dad was also a very talented artist and it was such a shame when he had to give this up because of the difficulty he had holding pastels between his fingers as the disease progressed.

Although I had won a colouring-in contest when I was seven, I didn't consider myself an artist in any way. I loved sewing and was quite clever with my hands. I could knit, crochet, do macramé and copper work as well as a bit of leatherwork. Then, after I'd moved to Bulahdelah in 2004, I decided to learn how to do folk art. I went to a local artist, Veronica Hughes and later, I went on to learn with some brilliant local artists, Ron and Helen Hindmarsh and I realised that I had in fact inherited some of my dad's talents in this field.

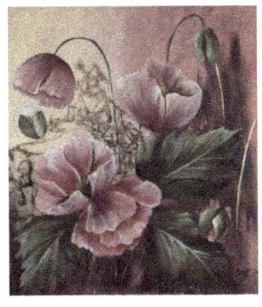
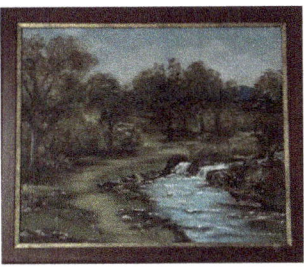
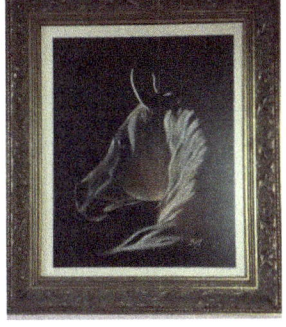

Three of my favourite paintings

My mum was a very special lady and I never really understood how truly special until I was much older. This is nothing unusual because as a child, you can only see things from a child's perspective. She protected us in so many ways and, looking back, always did things out of love. She expected us to behave well, have good manners and treat everyone the way we would like them to treat us.

She was tough in a different way. She had to independently learn to cope with being a wife and mother in a strange land, learning a completely foreign language and embracing new cultures and traditions.

The thing that really upset her was my father's non-acceptance of the three boys in our family. It's hard to believe any father could be like this but he was, and although everything looked quite rosy on the outside, beneath the surface, my older brothers and younger brother and I were quite badly scathed.

My younger sister, who is a lot like my dad, seemed to float through the experiences and was not aware of a lot of things that went on. There were many times when, because of something the boys had done, and because my mother defended the boys (and rightly so), my father would stop speaking to her and the boys – sometimes for up to six weeks (not a word).

During these times, he would sometimes speak nicely to me, not realising the dilemma this would always put me in. I loved my mum and 'hated' my father for what he put her through. I loved my brothers and 'hated' him for blaming them for things that were either normal for boys their age or unfair and misconstrued. I wanted to help my mum get through to him and make everything better. This taught me from a very early age that if things around me went wrong, it was up to me to make them right.

In her frustration, my mum would often say to me: 'Go and ask your father what I've done.'

Of course, he would never have an answer for me, because there was no answer. I could never understand how anyone could hold anger to this degree for so long and punish people they were supposed to love the way he did. I think this has always made me a lot more forgiving and I've often made excuses for other people's bad behaviour towards me and sometimes, I've been told, to the detriment of myself.

The most amazing thing though, was that out of the blue, my dad would wake up and everything would be back to normal, unless of course my mum started up with questions or expected an apology.

I can't imagine what my mum's life must have been like and the things she endured for so many years. She had no outlet, minimal real friends and very little money – the social security system was not as it is today.

Just before my 18th birthday, my parents had their first trip back to Holland for a few months. This was a gift from Mum's family. My eldest brother, Hans had long moved out of home and lived interstate, and my next brother, Sylvo had been living at home on and off (mostly off). My younger 14-year-old sister was at home, placed under my charge by my parents (I was 18 at the time), while my younger 10-year-old brother, Rene was with family friends.

As is often the case, families with emotional disturbances such as we experienced, produce children who try to deal with their problems in antisocial ways, including drug use.

Sylvo became reliant on drugs and was heavily into anything and everything. At this stage, he was using large quantities of heroin. Our family doctor had asked to see me and told me that if Sylvo didn't stop using drugs, he would be dead before the end of the year. At that time, I didn't write and tell my parents because they were on holidays and I didn't want to worry them. Besides, I believed it was my responsibility to look after him and to ensure that didn't happen. How naïve was I?

My parents returned from Holland mid-August and returned back to the reality of life.

In the beginning of September, Sylvo told Mum he was determined to kick his drug habit once and for all and had booked himself into the drug rehabilitation centre at Chermside Hospital.

My mum said a silent prayer of thanks because over the years she had had so much heartache and always felt so torn between her husband and her boys, knowing always that either she or the boys were the losers – there were no winners.

Father's Day started out with a great deal of tension because Dad was not talking to Mum and hadn't done so for at least a week.

We were very surprised when we heard a knock on the door early in the morning and saw our neighbor standing there looking quite uncomfortable. She asked if she could come in because she had some really bad news to tell Mum and Dad.

They sat her down in a chair and sat down themselves and then she said: 'I don't know how to tell you this, but I got a call from Chermside Hospital and they asked me if I could let you know that your son, Sylvo passed away during the night.'

The hospital had been given her number as contact person for Sylvo (at that time we couldn't afford a phone) hence, why they had rung her.

Imagine the shock.

Imagine the guilt.

Imagine the thoughts that must have gone through both their minds.

How could this have happened?

We would have celebrated with Sylvo his 21st birthday in two days' time. He would have had his whole life ahead of him ... and now it was gone ... never to be.

Naturally Mum and Dad and I wanted to know why he had died. This was not supposed to happen. The resultant autopsy showed he had died from a methadone overdose, plus he had endocarditis.

Given that this all happened in 1974 when there was a real stigma associated with drug addiction, parents were often given the blame and my mum had a real problem admitting she had a son who was drug addicted. She didn't want anyone to know he was getting treatment for this either, so we were all told to say he'd died from an asthma attack – which sounded reasonable and believable, given his past history.

The interesting and wonderful thing was, that although my dad was still never able to say sorry, he never again mistreated Mum by not speaking to her, and their relationship changed from that moment.

Sylvo's body was in the morgue in Chermside Hospital and needed to be formally identified. My mother was too distraught to do this, so she said I needed to go with my father and do it. It was the first time I'd seen a dead body and it wasn't the most pleasant thing I ever did.

At the time I had a lot of mixed, confused and angry feelings towards my mum, towards Sylvo, my brother and towards myself.

I had no one I could really talk to. I had no counselling. I had to pretend everything was okay. I had to carry on as normal and at the same time I was expected to act like I was grieving. I didn't know how I was expected to behave!

One night several weeks after Sylvo's death I went to a drive-in movie theatre with my boyfriend of over two years, Greg. As I was walking out the door, my mother started to rant and rave saying: 'That's the trouble with you! You have no feelings for anyone! Your brother is hardly dead and here you are, out having a good time as though nothing's happened! I've never known anyone so selfish!'

I rarely went out, and this evaluation of my actions was just not on. I wanted to tell her this was really unfair, but she really wasn't open to listening, so I kept my mouth shut, and although I still went out, it put a real dampener on my evening.

I started to have great difficulty with my own authenticity. I questioned everything in terms of how people might react to my actions, my words and in the end, my emotions. Showing my emotions became incongruent to what I was genuinely feeling at any given time. I often laughed when it wasn't appropriate, and this was quite embarrassing at times because I didn't know how I was expected to react.

I know now that my mum used me as a bit of a scapegoat for all of her misplaced grief and fortunately, we had the opportunity to talk about this well before her death and she was able to forgive herself and I was able to understand and forgive her as well.

Several years ago, Hans suggested we take Mum and Dad on a cruise to New Zealand on the Sea Princess. We knew it would not compare to Dad's past life of adventure on the high seas, but we hoped it would be a wonderful experience for him, and secretly we hoped it would mend the relationship Hans and he had, once and for all. Hans did say to me: 'I reckon we're both going to realise why we left home!'

My mother was quite severely affected by Alzheimer's at this time, although still living independently in a retirement village with my father. Although the four of us made plans together, mum had no recollection of any of these conversations.

As we were leaving Port Brisbane, she said to us: 'Where are we going?'
'We're going on a cruise to New Zealand just like we talked about – remember?' we reminded her.
'I don't remember anything of the sort,' she said, 'and I don't want to go!'

We decided to simply distract her and, as she was such a lover of nature, this was not a difficult thing to do.

As the cruise went on, she started to really love the cruising life. She was always happy and loved the interaction with all the staff, especially the waiters and cabin crew. She became quite well known on the ship because of her wonderful outgoing, loving nature and her willingness to participate in lots of things.

Dad was 90 years old when we did the cruise and we had difficulty getting travel insurance for him. Given his pre-existing medical conditions as well, a lot of things were excluded. This meant that we had to make sure he did not injure himself whilst on board. Although neither was wheelchair bound, we had two wheelchairs and both Mum and Dad sat in these going from place to place on the ship as well as whenever we did tours in the ports of New Zealand.

They had a suite and every night either Hans or I would stay on the fold-up divan so we could be there in case we were needed. They both needed assistance with showering and, depending on the roughness of the seas, with dressing for the day. This was where my dad became a bit truculent at times.

There were a number of incidents where his pride or stubbornness led to near falls and we needed to be hyper vigilant (and patient to the extreme) all the time.

On the ship, Mum really enjoyed the variety of food on the menu. She also loved the fun at mealtimes, enjoying the regular banter with the waiters and having the four of us together.

After dinner, they would go to the shows with Hans and I. Trevor, my husband joined our cruise halfway through as he'd been booked as one of the entertainers on board, so they got to see him as well. Both Mum and Dad were really big fans.

In the Atrium, playing piano and entertaining the crowd (which seemed to grow every night) was a great entertainer, Dave (Piano-man) Johnson. Thankfully, my dad really liked listening to him, because this meant he would want to go there every night.

My mum just loved it because it gave her a chance to dance. She had always loved dancing and used to reminisce about it regularly, but Dad would never dance with her. Obviously in later years he couldn't, but Hans took her onto the dance floor and together they laughed, and you could see her just glowing as this part of her came to life. She had terrible corns on her feet as well as hammertoes, but none of this stopped her.

Towards the end of the cruise, she got to know her way back to her cabin and would say she was going back to her 'little house'.

So many people used to come up to Hans and I and comment on how wonderful we were with our parents. They said what a pleasure it was to see the love between us and our parents and how selfless we were in doing this. Some went as far as to say they wished they had children like us. Little did they know that for us it was just as wonderful, and we got so much satisfaction from seeing Mum come to life the way she did and to see the sparkle in her eyes and to enjoy and get to see Dad in a new light as well.

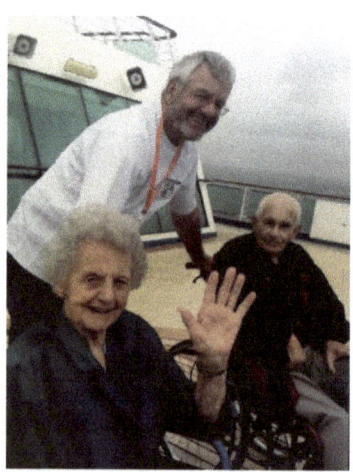

Hans, with Mum and Dad on our cruise.

Both Hans and I have such fond memories of this wonderful time and we got to see Mum the way Dad must have seen her years ago when he first fell in love with her. We realised the strong connection and love they had for each other – one that held them together through thick and thin and through all of life's ups and downs of their lives together.

As I grew into adulthood and beyond, I developed a really strong connection with both Mum and Dad and am forever grateful that I was able to see Dad for who he really was and to be there with him and make a difference in his final lucid hours.

Although I wasn't able to be there in person with my mum when she died, she died a very peaceful death in the presence of her three children, Hans, Ingrid and Rene, as well as their spouses and grandchildren, three years after Dad died.

She had Alzheimer's for a number of years prior to her death and this changed her. In our formative years, especially as we were growing up, she was highly anxious (understandably so, due to the fact she was walking on eggshells most of the time). In later years, she and Dad travelled extensively around Australia. They both loved being in nature and loved classical music and they loved each other very much.

Towards the end with every accumulative year, Mum became more loving and more expressive of this love.

I was living in Bulahdelah, New South Wales and she was in Prins Willem Alexander Nursing Home in Birkdale, Queensland and I remember whenever I would come to visit, her face would just light up. It was only at the very end that she didn't recognise us anymore, but this never stopped her showing her gratitude to us for visiting her and we always noticed that, with regular visits, she was more interactive, cognisant and seemed happier.

I remember talking to her once after we'd returned from our cruise, about a problem I had with one of my children, and she said: 'Just love them, Maya, and let them know you love them. Accept that they have to live their own lives and that they will make mistakes. Never be afraid to say sorry and always be there for them when they need you.'

During the latter years of my mum's life, I got so much of the nurturing and hugs and cuddles I missed out on as a child. It is so important to get these in your formative years, and I realise all too well how differently I would have seen myself had I gotten this then, and throughout my life. However, as with most things, there are no regrets, only experiences that have contributed into making me who I am today.

'Miracle in Richards Bay - Escape from the Vortex' by Maya Knight

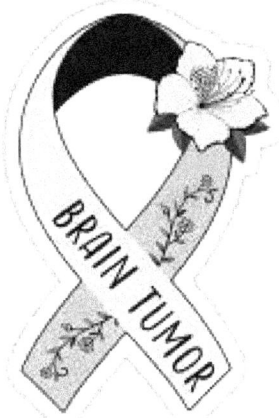

When you focus
On the narrative of your life,
You become bogged down
In the tiny details and forget the ripples
That change the tides of time
And change your life.

Life is a journey
And you meet many on your path
Some you see as obstacles,
Not realising their true worth
In the order of things.
You must always remember
All that you have learned from them
And all you have become because of them.

CHAPTER 4

It was at a credit union dinner dance when I was 16, that I met Greg Jones, the boy who was to become my first husband. He was there with his father and I was there with my parents. We had a really lovely evening, getting to know each other and dancing closely together. Both of us were quite innocent and our friendship blossomed into a relationship over the next four years.

His father was my father's boss and also a member on the board, and although this might have complicated our relationship, it didn't. His dad was really happy that Greg had found such a lovely girl and he did everything in his power to make sure his son had opportunities to see me. The big problem we had was that Greg's mother was totally against Greg meeting up with any girl and totally disapproved of me (sight unseen). As you can imagine, this totally fed into, and solidified my belief even further, that I wasn't good enough.

Obviously, his mother did come to approve of me, but that only happened because of an almighty row between her and Greg's dad.

Before this, I think his dad had just resigned himself to living this horrid existence of not being appreciated and being dictated to and I think it took this for him to finally find the strength to leave her and find some happiness for himself.

I know it was a difficult decision for him and he did pay a high price because his now ex-wife spent years poisoning their then 10-year-old daughter's mind. Fortunately, although a lot of this damage is often irreparable, he and Greg's sister did reunite and build a strong relationship when she was in her late teens.

Greg and I were there for him throughout this time and he came to depend a lot on me for support throughout the years that followed, even after his son and I separated and divorced. I learned from this that I needed to be responsible and be there for others when they needed someone.

When I was 19, Greg and I went for a trip to the Snowy Mountains. My mother was aghast because she was a real believer that I should remain 'pure' until I was married. On that trip, we announced our engagement and were married three months later.

It was easy for me to settle into married life because we already had a good friendship and rarely argued.

At age 24, I gave birth to my beautiful baby girl, Kristy. I thought my life would be complete with a baby, but obviously she hadn't read the book!

After a 60-hour labour, haemorrhoids, Greg's grandfather's death (the day after her birth), five months of colic, lots of advice from well-meaning family and friends, I was not only exhausted, but reached the conclusion I was a bad mother. Obviously, I couldn't talk to anyone about this, not even Greg. I felt shame and told myself I just had to try harder.

At this stage we had saved really hard, had a beautiful house, two golden retriever dogs and life should have been great, but it wasn't, and the reason was because of how I felt about myself.

I decided to go back to work (after a year off) but that really didn't help much either, because my parents disapproved of working mothers and would let me know all too often what a disappointment I was to them.

My younger sister, who'd broken all their rules as she was growing up, was now married and living 'respectably' in her very routine life – unlike me! Over the years, I was to be reminded of the big differences between us, and how I just didn't measure up in their eyes.

When Kristy was five, her dad and I split up. Knowing how traumatic this can be for children, I wanted the impact to be as minimal as possible upon Kristy. Greg was a good man. It was just that we were better as friends than as husband and wife.

Greg and I mutually decided not to have solicitors involved and came to a financial agreement that benefitted both our lifestyles at the time. We had an arrangement that he would come to the house for dinner every Wednesday so he could have some time with Kristy, and he had also requested to have her every weekend.

Obviously, this arrangement left a bit to be desired and I hadn't really thought it through.

I began to feel used as he started to expect a good meal and then just go off with Kristy for his play-time with her. Not once did he help me with the dishes or cleaning up!
The straw that broke the camel's back came when he told me he wouldn't be able to see Kristy as often because …'I have a life of my own, you know.'

I told him to explain this to her, which of course he didn't, and, as time went by and his life became fuller, with other women, their children, his interests and a move interstate, his visits became more and more infrequent.

She felt abandoned by him and in the absence of a good explanation, she blamed me – after all, if I hadn't been on his case, he would want to come around more, which she translated to, being with her more often.

She always felt she had to protect him and there was nothing I could really say or do to change this. I certainly didn't want to blacken his name in any way and he really was a good man, and loved her very much, despite our differences.

As a single mum, I had a lot of financial and emotional responsibilities. I believe in teaching my children good manners and creating a person who is kind, responsible for their own behaviour and able to function independently and leave a positive mark on others. We had some great times together, but I must admit at times the pressures of life and doing it all alone really got the better of me. My family tended to believe that 'if you make your bed, you must lie in it!' so they were not really forthcoming with any real support – financial or emotional.

I was very committed to motherhood and although I had a bit of a social life, I kept it to a minimum because there just wasn't the time, and I didn't want anything to compromise my responsibility towards Kristy. Besides, I really loved my times together with Kristy and I enjoyed watching her grow up.

Some years later at a vulnerable time in my life, I met my second husband, Peter.

Peter was besotted with me and couldn't get enough of me. This of course fed my low opinion of myself and before I knew it, I had agreed to marry him. I would like to say this was the biggest regret in my life but how can I do so when my son, Steven was the result?

I was deceived very early on in this relationship and had no experience of the cruelty of some human beings. I took him for better or worse and believe me, he turned out much worse than what I took him for.

After we married, Peter became the proprietor of our local Residential Real Estate Agency (something he'd never done before). The expectation was that I was to work in it with him and I did so, putting in long hours, which as it turned out, were pretty much for nothing, because in the end we lost all our money and property.

We were together 24 hours a day, most days, and although there were some good times, the bad times far outweighed these.

He took delight in frightening me and emotionally and physically tormenting me. I understood what it felt like to be abused, to feel unsafe and mostly, I understood the lengths I was prepared to go so my children were protected and safe.

I had a new-formed respect for the plight of abused women and really understood why so many remain silent. All too often, it's the safest option.

I learned to be scared when I was with him and more scared when I didn't know where he was, because I knew he was prepared to stop at nothing to bring me down.

He tried to discredit me in the workplace and threatened everyone I loved, as well as the things I treasured.

I couldn't talk to anyone about it, because those I did were very quick to judge me and very quick to give me their opinion and simple advice: 'If it's so bad, why don't you leave him?'

So easy to say ... not so easy to do.

I spent time in a women's refuge, and I looked at many options – most of them futile.

I was one of the lucky ones though, because due to circumstances, Peter moved 1,000kilometres away, back in with his parents in Townsville, taking his then-12-year-old son with him.

I was left to cope with no income, impending bankruptcy, two children to support (Kristy, who was now 11 years old and my beautiful baby boy, Steven who wasn't even a year old), a car that was being repossessed and a house I had to pack up and move out of within two weeks.

And I did it because I had to and because my children were depending on me.

Life moved on and things started to get back into a normal, happy routine. I remember so many great times with Kristy, Steven and myself. We went for drives, to the park and we always found ways on a limited budget to enjoy and appreciate each other and what we had. We had regular contact with family and some friends and life was good.

Kristy was growing up fast and sport was a huge focus for her. She loved anything competitive. This competitive spirit has stayed with her throughout her entire life, making her resilient and a truly formidable opponent to the challenges in life.

My son, Steven was 10 years her junior and it always seemed like I had two 'only' children. He was such a cute little boy and as he grew older, he always had a real softness and gentleness to his nature.

I count my blessings knowing that despite all the hardships and mistakes I made over the years, I have raised two wonderful human beings who bring such joy and love into my life and the lives of others. I am so proud of them and all they have achieved.

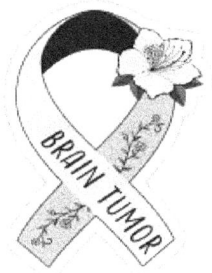

Believe in unconditional love
For there are no other meanings
For love.

If you live with love
As your one and only signpost
Along the maze of indecisions
And travails in your life,
You will indeed be remunerated
And live a true, full and abundant life.

Love is the peace that comes
When you behold the beauty in yourself,
In everyone around you,
And in the environment
You live in.

CHAPTER 5

It's amazing how the Universe can catapult you to be exactly where it wants you to be, and what can be even more amazing is the timing.

It was the beginning of 2002 and I had been working long hours and really needed a break.

As a result, I had booked a three-day cruise. This would be the first holiday I'd had in ages and the first holiday I had without my children. I rarely took any time off and always saved my sick leave. I did this just in case there was a time I might really need it, for example, if something unforeseen happened to my children.

However, fate had other plans. As it happened, the cruise line had overbooked, and my booking wasn't registering.

Imagine my disappointment.

At this time, Kristy was in her early 20s, and was living with me temporarily. She had had her first baby, Jaydn and he was such a delight.

When she saw how disappointed I was, she talked me into taking a real holiday – not just a three-day getaway. She suggested I take a decent time away going to somewhere I really wanted to go. She even made it sound like I was doing her the favour, rather than the other way around. So off I went, leaving Steven in her very capable hands.

On May 3, 2002, I boarded the Pacific Sky cruise ship not realising from that moment on, my life would never be the same again.

I was directed to my cabin, one I shared with three other women. In those days, prior to the tragic Dianne Brimble case, if you asked to share a four-berth stateroom, the cruise line would make all the arrangements to try to match you up with people the same age and sex as you. This was the cheapest way to have a holiday.

I couldn't believe I was here!

For the next 10 days, I looked forward to being pampered at sea and having no responsibilities. We were going to New Zealand, somewhere I'd always wanted to go but never thought I would. There was so much I planned to see and do, and due to fabulous weather throughout the trip, I got to see everything I had on my to do, see and experience list.

New Zealand was the most amazing place with the most breathtaking scenery at every turn. It was only the people who surpassed it. I couldn't believe how friendly they all were. Asking someone for directions usually included them actually escorting you there. I just loved the genuineness and kindness of the New Zealanders.

Life on board was just jam-packed with entertainment from dawn until the early hours of the morning, and then some. Not being one for drinking or the nightclub scene, I tended to enjoy the more sedate entertainment. I loved trivia and I really loved the big shows in the auditoriums.

There was a male entertainer who did several performances, mostly due to popular requests from the passengers – and I could see why. I went to all his shows and even doubled up on some just to hear him again. I bought one of his CDs in the shop on board. We were only halfway through the cruise and he'd already sold out, so that was the only reason I didn't buy more. 'Just my luck,' I thought.

He had the most amazing voice and could play the guitar like no other. He did John Denver's songs, as well as some covers and some originals. I couldn't believe how talented he was; I could have listened to him for hours.

Never in my wildest dreams would I have imagined this man would become my third husband – but as they say, third time lucky!

I remember how we met as though it were yesterday.

I had decided to go to karaoke with one of my roommates. However, as we were in the lift going to the 10th floor, something possessed me and I pressed the button in the lift to the seventh floor and said to her: 'Let's check out the Verandah Bar.'

I think she thought I was mad because we were already late, and this stopover would make us even later.

I said to her: 'Let's sit here,' which we did, and within minutes, Trevor Knight, the amazing performer I'd drooled over, walked over to me. He looked directly into my eyes and said: 'I don't dance, but would you like to?'

'Would I like to . . . Is the Pope Catholic? Of course I'd like to!'

We had several slow dances and magic happened. I didn't want to open my eyes in case I was dreaming. This sort of thing couldn't be happening to me.

He then asked me if I'd like to go up to the cocktail bar, where it was a little quieter and we could talk. My roommate started to tag along initially but I suggested she might prefer karaoke. Thank goodness she took the hint.

Little did I know that a few days prior to this, Trevor had done a small intimate show and I had requested he sing *Goodbye Again* and he obliged. Straight after that, I went to see a movie I'd wanted to see for a long time, so I left. However, he didn't know this and was looking around for 'the voice'. He told me later that he'd spent days chatting up women just to see if the voice matched the one he'd heard requesting *Goodbye Again*, and of course it didn't, until he heard me speak.

The other interesting thing was, that at the precise time I went to the Verandah Bar, he had put the key in the lock of his stateroom because he was about to watch a film he'd been intent on watching for ages when a little voice said: 'Go to the Verandah Bar.' So, for no logical reason, he took the key out of the lock and proceeded up to the Verandah Bar. He told me he had no idea why he'd done this because he never goes to bars.

The following day, we met up and I told him I was a palmist. Well, this really interested him and as is so often the case, he asked: 'Can you read my hands?'

Unbeknown to him, I really wanted to read them because then I could see all his character traits, especially the ones that often don't surface until well into a relationship.

I'd made so many poor judgments in the past and I really didn't want to go down that track again.

He had really interesting hands and had a Simian line on his right hand. This is one straight line that encompasses both the heart and head lines; it begins halfway between the thumb and index finger and goes horizontally straight across the palm. He had the usual heart and head-lines on his left hand. This indicated to me that he liked to keep his work and private lives separate but, when involved in something, could become almost obsessed to the point of ignoring anyone and everything else. I wondered if I would be able to cope with this, and I decided that I would need to be mindful of this as a character trait and therefore not take it as a personal affront. As it turned out, his ability to do this has been the reason for his success in so many areas where others have failed. There were many other signs obviously and I was so impressed with 'who' I really saw before me that I decided I would go where fate took me.

But, where were things going to go from here?

He lived in Berry, NSW and I lived in Edens Landing, Brisbane, Queensland.

Also, he was off on another land tour in New Zealand and I was flying home from Auckland the following day.

We both had completely different lives and I really thought this was just a nice shipboard romance.

However, in the back of my mind I thought: 'The Universe has gone to such extraordinary lengths to get us together and I really believed there was a reason for this, even though I didn't know it at the time.'

After I returned home, a friend of mine was visiting me and she suggested I invite myself to his place.

'I can't do that,' I said. 'What on earth will he think of me? Besides, I have Steven to think of.'

As the days went by though, I couldn't get him out of my mind. I don't know what possessed me, but I rang and asked if he'd like me to come down to Berry for a few days. Now if that wasn't forward enough, on our trip down to his farm, I said: 'I don't know why, but I just have to tell you that I love you!'

He stopped the car and said: 'That's exactly how I feel about you.'

We had only known each other two days on the ship and another eight days where we had contacted each other by email or phone. It was ridiculous and I couldn't explain it. It was like it was so totally out of character for me, but I felt more like 'me' than I'd ever felt in my life.

Trevor had booked a trip to England several months prior to him meeting me and he was due to go a few days after I left his farm and went back home.

For some reason I felt confident enough in this relationship to say to him that if he wanted another relationship with someone, then that was fine with me, as long as he knew that it would spell the end of our relationship. I was never ever going to play second fiddle again.

While he was on his way to England to visit his mum and family he suddenly thought: 'What am I doing? I'm going the wrong way!'

As soon as he landed, he booked a return ticket to Sydney, but he had to stay in England for four days before he could head back home to me.

As soon as he landed back in Sydney, he picked up his car and drove up to Brisbane. He was so tired after a mammoth flight that he just had to find a motel and rest, and of all places, he stopped at The Lady Jane Motel in Bulahdelah (for any of you who drive past, they make the best pizzas).

Little did we know then that this would be the place we'd end up living.

Of course, I was totally unprepared for a visit and one at such short notice.

I was still working fulltime, so when he first arrived, it was Kristy who met him at the door and entertained him until I got home a few hours later.

He stayed a month and we realised how magical our connection was. We often didn't need words because we seemed to know what the other was thinking.

In the week before he went back to Berry, he suggested we have a special night out, so we went to this wonderful seafood restaurant in South Bank, on the banks of the Brisbane River where World Expo had been held in 1988.

It was a lovely evening in June and the weather was still pleasant, so we chose to sit outdoors by a fire. As we were waiting for our meal to arrive, he said: 'I want to ask you something. Will you marry me?'

You could have knocked me over with a feather. We had discussed marriage prior to this and, given my track record and his views that marriage wasn't important, I was flabbergasted!

Then it was like something bore deep into my solar plexus and I heard a voice say: 'Isn't this what you want?'

So, I told him I'd think about it ... only I couldn't hold him in suspense for too long because I knew this was truly what I'd been waiting for my whole life.

He went home and we agreed I'd go down to Berry and live there with him. If you'd asked me then, I would have said: 'I'd given up so much for him', but if you asked me today, that answer would be different. He has added to my life in so many ways and each day I count my blessings that he is beside me in this journey we call our life, sharing the ups and downs, the joys and heartbreaks and always with the deepest love, trust and respect for each other.

Now I could say that he was just too good to be true and he was my perfect match and that would be the truth, but it would be the Mills &Boon version of the truth.

The reality is that every relationship is made up of two separate individuals with their own personality, habits and baggage. It's about understanding 'who' the other person really is and being able to accept them as they are, without wanting to change them.

More importantly though, it's about being able to be yourself, wholly and completely.

It's about knowing that you don't complete the other person, but that the relationship allows you to grow into the complete person that you are.

This was what our relationship was like.

We married on January 3, 2003 and lived in Berry, Trevor's old stamping ground, for 18 months. Neither of us had any money to speak of because we hadn't made any demands from our ex-spouses and had both lost a lot in the process of our divorces.

My parents' opinions had always been quite important to me as they are to most children (despite their age) and I remember clearly when they visited Trevor and me when we were still living in Berry.

Mum had previously said to me that she would never really accept any man other than my first husband, Greg as my one true spouse. However, on seeing Trevor and I together and seeing the way he treated me and the love we had together, she said to me: 'Maya, I was wrong. I can see now that this is the man you belong with.'

This was a special moment for me, and I really appreciated that she could see this and that she had told me.

For the first few years of our lives together, Trevor did a lot more cruising than I did. He had been working as an entertainer for many years and started getting more and more contracts on the Princess line.

This meant that he would fly out to catch a ship in different countries around the world in an overseas port and disembark in an overseas port as well.
At this stage, Steven, my son, was still a child and obviously I needed to be home with him in these formative years.

We'd been living in Berry together for 18 months when we decided to relocate so we could both have a new beginning.

However, we had a long list of requirements that would need to be met.

We needed to be somewhere that was close enough to Sydney for Trevor to continue working in the larger clubs and venues and continue cruising. We needed to be close to a hospital with a psychiatric ward for me to continue my nursing. We needed a large block of land for our horses, cows, donkeys and dogs and we needed a reasonable house that we could live in and enjoy.

This was easier said than done, because at the time, we could only afford to rent and we found very early on, that this would be nigh on impossible to find.

I suggested we do a Dream Board. The three of us then spent a few days choosing pictures and words that represented what we wanted in our new home and these were pasted onto a piece of cardboard and placed in a prominent place where we could see it several times a day.

Nothing happened at first and then, when we went into Berry to buy some groceries, I told Trevor that we needed to buy 'The Land' newspaper. As it was a Sunday, he said we should wait until the following Thursday when the new edition came out, but I was insistent, saying: 'No! There's something in this one for us.'

As we got home, I opened it up and right at the page I opened, there was a four-bedroom house for rent in a place called Bulahdelah on a 70-acre property.

We had no idea where Bulahdelah was, despite Trevor having stopped there when he'd come to see me in Brisbane for that first fateful time. Given the sound of the name, we thought it was out in the back of beyond, somewhere way outback in the middle of nowhere. The rent sounded reasonable, so we thought we'd give them a call.

We were really surprised to hear that it was just north of Newcastle on the main Pacific Highway. We asked the owners if we could arrange to come and see the property and if they would hold it for us until we had; and they agreed.

We were on our way up to Brisbane for one of Trevor's tours the following Saturday, so arranged to see it the day before.

After coming to the quaint old town of Bulahdelah, we turned onto the Old Pacific Highway, then turned onto a dirt road in the middle of a national park and drove onto the property.

Trevor took one look and said: 'We're not leaving until they agree that we can have it.'

We drove down the driveway and met the owners and I think they were as taken with us as we were with them. They were really wonderful country folk and there and then we made arrangements for when we would move in.

When we got back to Berry and looked at our Dream Board, it ticked every single box.

After a few years, the owners wanted to sell and as agreed, they gave us first right of refusal. We moved Heaven and Earth and managed to get a hefty deposit and a bank mortgage and acquired what we call *Our Little Piece of Heaven*.

When Steven became more independent, I got the opportunity to go with Trevor on some more of the P&O cruises because these were usually round trips from Sydney and return. I really loved the cruising lifestyle and I regularly did talks on palmistry on the ships.

As time went by, Princess Cruises heard what I did and recognised my value, adding me to Trevor's contracts and we became a double act, with me offering lectures and workshops. Trevor also started doing lectures and workshops as well as extra shows on top of the mandatory night-time main shows.

Princess Cruises have been very generous to both of us over the years and always looked after us as we travelled to various destinations throughout the world.

It's been so rewarding when passengers have been thrilled to see we are booked on their cruise, because they know we have a large, varied repertoire of entertainment. We have made so many lifelong friends and amassed so many wonderful memories over the years.

It wasn't always easy for me as a suburban girl, getting used to living in the country. There were so many things to get used to, but over the years, we have created the most wonderful home and life together.

Although our children are all grown up now and living away from home, we have added to our family with the horses we breed and Willow's Whippets, our wonderful sought-after whippet puppies.

'Miracle in Richards Bay - Escape from the Vortex' by Maya Knight

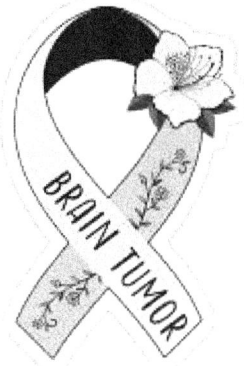

Hardships come to you
In order that you may reach
Deep into your soul
For that which lies deep within.

It is through struggles that
You come to a greater understanding
Of yourself.

Look forward into the unknown
Knowing with certainty
That within 'you' lies the strength
To face all that may come.

CHAPTER 6

February 3-9

I woke up on the morning of February 3, 2020 feeling really excited because we were flying to Sri Lanka where we'd been contracted to join the Sun Princess on her exotic itinerary to The Seychelles, Zanzibar, Nosy Be in Madagascar and Richards Bay (Zululand) from where we'd cruise around the coast of South Africa, then on to Cape Town from where we would disembark and fly home.

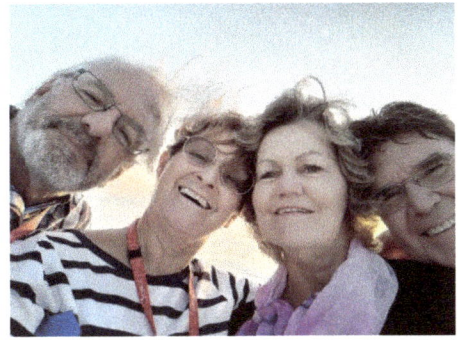

Hans, Rowena, Trevor and me a few days prior to me being hospitalised on board.

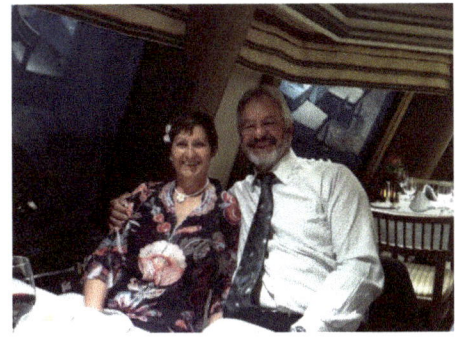

Hans and Rowena enjoying the cruising lifestyle.

We were also meeting up with my brother, Hans and his wife, Rowena who were doing the full cruise.

We had three weeks of meeting new people, catching up with people we'd met before, being totally spoiled by the wonderful crew on board and enjoying the entertainment, fun and food.

I'd never been to Sri Lanka before and was a bit disappointed that we wouldn't really get a chance to see the city because we arrived in the evening and would be going straight to our hotel and then being picked up early the following morning and taken to the ship.

The hotel was an hour's drive from the airport but it felt like it was never going to end. This was one of the most harrowing experiences in my life.

I'd heard about the chaos on the roads in India and Vietnam, but personally I didn't have much personal experience of this because I'd never been there.

It was a bit of a blur of car horns, putt-putts, tyres squealing, brakes screeching. Even though it was a public holiday and eight o'clock at night, with not as much traffic as usual, I got to realise very quickly, that in Sri Lanka, the car horn takes the place of literally everything. Our driver used it instead of braking, instead of indicating and as well as acknowledging other drivers he knew. He wove in and out of traffic, never bothering to slow down and rarely braking. To help him out, I nearly wore through the floor of the car in the back seat where we sat, as I kept pushing down on the brake pedal that of course wasn't there.

I don't know how we got there in one piece and it amazes me how their vehicles don't sustain more damage than they do. I felt like a cat that had just used up one of its nine lives.

After a good night's sleep, we went to the port and went through the embarkation process.

It always amazes me how travelling changes your perception of time. For a start, being in another country means that you have to be aware of the different time zones and that a person on the other side of the world can either be in your tomorrow or your yesterday.

The other thing that always amazes me is that whenever we have a break from cruising and then get back on a ship, it's as though we never left, and we just take up where we left off.

The same applies when we get home. It's like the time on board the ship never existed, and life goes on as before.

So, there we were, back on the wonderful Sun Princess, one of our favourite ships, really looking forward to the next few weeks. We had so many things we planned to do – lots of lectures, workshops and shows.

We had no idea that this would all be cut short and that our lives and the way of the world would never be the same again.

February 9-14

"Birth ... Death and everything in between is life."

This was the introduction to my first talk, *Your Life is in Your Hands*, to an audience of a few hundred people – an interactive talk where I invite people to look at certain aspects of their hands and I tell them what it describes about them as a person.

However, I was not long into the talk when I started struggling for words and seemed to lose my train of thought. I watched some people leave (never a good sign) but I really couldn't blame them, as I was fumbling for words and giving a performance far below my usual standard and also far below an acceptable standard.

'What's wrong with me?' I thought.

I carried on as best I could, going in and out of this vagueness and losing my lucidity as well as my ability to put my thoughts together in a logical way. I was quite aware of the mish-mash I was making of things and I avoided making eye contact with Trevor or Hans, my brother because I knew I would have some explaining to do after I'd finished.

I really felt embarrassed, and I had no logical explanation for what had just happened.

As I expected, Trevor asked me what was wrong, and if I was alright – he'd never seen me lose it like I'd just done. This actually made me feel worse than I already did, as there was nothing I could say to explain what had just happened. They said they noticed me looking really flustered and vague at times and that I seemed to be struggling with bigger words and concepts.

I felt like crying and I just wanted to flee the scene of my disgrace.

However, it wasn't going to be that easy because several people who'd seen me do my shows before came down to where I was and asked me if I was okay or if I was nervous, because they had certainly noticed a big difference in my performance from the last time they'd seen me and knew something was wrong. They were being really supportive, each in their own way and I did realise this at the time, but it just highlighted to me how bad a performance I'd given.

I was really close to tears and was fighting to keep them at bay, finding it so much harder to do with all these people showing me such compassion, understanding, kindness and basically being really nice to me. The sad thing though, was I had no words for anyone – no reason and no explanation for my out-of-character behaviour.

Both Hans and Trevor commended me for continuing on and said they didn't know whether they could have. This was a bit of a back-handed compliment – was I really *that* bad?

I knew there was something not quite right in the way I was thinking, and I asked Trevor to speak to our wonderful cruise director, Ruth, and ask her if she could excuse me from doing any more lectures or workshops. I was really afraid it could happen again. He told her I wasn't feeling well. Thank goodness she was amenable.

She had come by during my talk to see the attendance and to see how things were going and had arrived at a time when I was doing well. Seeing I had a full auditorium, she was really pleased and had no idea of the disaster that had occurred before and after she'd been there. Part of her job requires her to fill in reports on all the guest lecturers and entertainers so Princess Cruises can continue to give their passengers the high calibre of entertainment they have come to expect.

One lady who saw me in passing prior to me doing my show, said she was so thrilled that I was on the ship because she had seen me before, had had a reading and had been blown away by how accurate it had been. She hadn't known how to get back in contact with me, so when she saw I was on board, she told her friend and they both wanted to book in to see me. I got her details and said I'd phone her in her stateroom and we could make arrangements.

I phoned her room the day after my show and her husband answered the phone. Again, out of the blue, I couldn't get my words out. I couldn't even let him know that it was me ringing. That afternoon after a nanna-nap I decided I would try again. After all it was probably due to the fact that I was tired, so I tried again. No one answered but there was an option to leave a message. I got flustered … what was I supposed to say?

I couldn't think, so I just hung up. Trevor suggested I write down what I wanted to say and read it out. However, this didn't work either because I got stuck between reading and being able to project the words as intelligible speech. I just could not do it, no matter how hard I tried. In the end, I gave up.

I felt defeated. I felt useless because I couldn't fulfill this small task and I didn't know why. I knew at this stage there was no way I would be able to engage in any meaningful two-way conversation with a stranger because it might just happen again, so I chose to just retreat into myself. I decided to distance myself from the passengers wherever possible. This was the only safe option for me. Everything else came with its own consequences, which, at that stage, I was not up to addressing. I didn't see this woman again on the ship and hopefully one day our paths will cross again, and she will understand.

As the days went by, although I could still understand everything, my ability to speak logically and in full sentences started diminishing even more. I was finding it hard to think clearly as well.

I remember looking at Trevor as he was working out his *There's a Song in Your Heart* songwriting workshop and just wondering how he could be so creative and switch his mind from one thing to another. I had never had any trouble in the past switching from one thing to another, from one thought to another, but I just couldn't do it now. It was like I was an observer of everything around me.

I was only able to hold one thought at a time and I certainly had lost my ability to multitask. It felt a bit like I was just tagging along for the ride and, not only had I lost my voice literally, I had also lost any inkling of having a voice. This was something that would surprise those who know me well, because I do like to be heard; I do like to have a point of view and I do like to express it.

I was turning into a *Stepford Wife* (the idyllic version of the perfect wife who just goes along with anything and everything and never rocks the boat ... and very happy to do so).

For me though ... what other choice did I have?

The strange thing was that most of the time I wasn't even that concerned, nor was I concerned about what was happening to me. I just kept thinking I'd wake up and be back to normal.

Between my brother, Hans, his wife, Rowena and me, we had a wealth of information at our disposal with Rowena having a general nursing background, Hans and I having psychiatric nursing backgrounds, Hans having a health, social work background in neurosurgery and neurology – all to very qualified levels I might add. Also, Trevor is highly intelligent and lived a full life where he'd learned a lot about physiology (horses mainly) and various medical implications. His son is a pathologist, and his daughter is a veterinary specialist, so, as a group, we had speculated as to what was wrong with me on several occasions.

Later Hans and Rowena did say they had had grave concerns for me, and had several conversations, wondering if what was wrong with me was just functional or something more sinister. Was it nerves? Was it that I hadn't done my talk for some time? Was it that I was tired – after all, I had been working in my nursing job, sometimes doing eighteen-hour shifts in the weeks prior to coming on the cruise? Or was there actually something organically/physically wrong with my brain causing these symptoms? As they said later, it was much safer to think that the cause may have been functional rather than something organic, like a stroke or a brain tumour.

They figured that without proper tests, it was difficult to make any assumptions, and being very considerate of my feelings at the time, they felt they were there to support me, rather than pressure me and add to any anxiety I might be feeling. They knew that, for the most part, I understood everything clearly, but couldn't express myself. They also believed that I retained the capacity to make my own decisions and I would ask for help if I needed it. I knew they would be there for me on whatever level I was comfortable with or needed, and that was really comforting for me.

I felt so blessed to have them there because they normalised things for me as much as possible. We shared a lot of our meals and watched the shows together. In lots of ways, they protected me from others knowing that something was wrong with me.

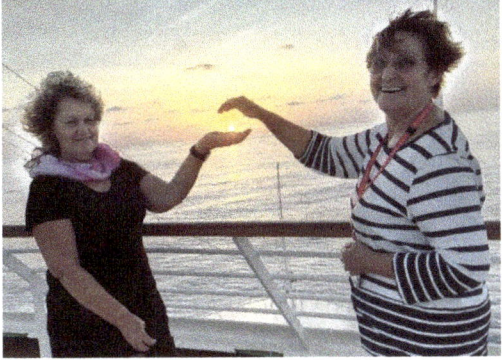

Rowena and I used to go for walks around the decks. Here we are 'catching the last bit of sun'.

Rowena and I went for long walks up and down stairs and around the promenade deck, with her chatting as I listened. Occasionally though, I was able to interject with a few words. This was really wonderful – enjoying the majestic Sun Princess as it ploughed its way seamlessly through the Indian Ocean.

All the while we wondered: 'What would the workers of the world be doing right now, while we're relaxing and enjoying life?'

We were very lucky on this particular cruise because Trevor and I were also able to be tour escorts. In doing this, we got to go on shore tours with the passengers with the only payment being to offer assistance if required. Afterwards, we would do a written report. It was rare to put two tour guides on a bus together and we knew this. Although we could put in first, second and third preferences for which tours we wanted to go on, we didn't find out until the night before which ones they'd booked for us (if any). We enjoyed going on separate tours though, because afterwards we would compare photos and experiences with each other. It almost doubled our experience of our port of call.

The first shore excursion was *The Seychelles* and, although Trevor and I were on separate buses, we were on the same trip, going to the same places, although our times at different highlights of the trip were staggered. However, it meant that we stopped at the same place and time for lunch. As soon as I got off the bus, I looked out for Trevor and spotted him with a group of passengers from his bus. Thankfully, he had saved a seat for me at one of the tables. He introduced me to all of them and at this stage I was still able to make a little bit of small talk. Trevor saved my bacon several times by holding court, so no one really noticed there was anything wrong with me. They just thought I was quiet.

Lunch was a smorgasbord of delectable island fare – beautiful salads, fruits and whole carved fish and meats as well as sumptuous pasta dishes. It makes my mouth water just thinking back on this.

I remember the flooring of the restaurant – just beautiful fine sand. This was such a wonderful sensation, especially after being on board. I just love the feeling of talcum powder, soft sand between my toes. In fact, I really didn't want to put my shoes back on. Naturally, the kitchen area was designed differently, for health and safety reasons.

The Seychelles is a very special place for me. It's where some of my special memories live. I reminisced too, when we'd flown here a year ago and were taken to a hotel on the other side of the island prior to embarking the Pacific Princess the following day. We'd been picked up by our driver and had travelled up similar mountainous, lush peaks. The roads were very narrow. It astounded me that more cars weren't swallowed up by the huge gutters, waterways and drainage systems on both sides of the roads. I'm sure it was directly as a result of channeling water down the mountains this way that kept these roads in such good condition. When we'd arrived at our motel, it took our breath away.

We'd had our honeymoon on this ship 17 years ago and this place, looking over the sea, felt like a honeymoon all over again. We went for walks along the beach in the moonlight and again early the next morning. To say it was magical was an understatement.

And here we were again on this lush, pristine island, even though we were on the other side of it this time. We both still felt the magical appeal and were still captivated by the natural, island feel, especially with the noise of the waves on the rocks in the background, the contrasts between high mountain tops and pristine shorelines, the magnificent views and the plentiful songs of the birds that inhabited the skies and nested in the trees.

After our lunch, which some lingered over longer than others, we could choose to walk by the ocean if we wanted to, or to see the huge tortoises that were together in an enclosure just outside the restaurant. This area housed about eight huge tortoises (we never did get to ask how old they were) and they seemed very happy with lots of food and plenty of shelter and room to move. They were fully enclosed so we could all walk around the perimeter in the hope that one or more would come to the edge to say hello.

Trevor is really good with animals and is well known for his natural horsemanship abilities. However, I didn't think for a minute that this translated to these beautiful creatures as well. The other passengers around the enclosure were trying to entice the tortoises over closer to them so they could give them a scratch, but none of the tortoises seemed interested.

However, Trevor put his hand over the three-foot high fence and offered one of them some of the leaves in there that was their food, and lo and behold, this tortoise came up really close to him, and then started lifting his head right up so Trevor could give him a scratch.

Other tortoises started doing the same, clambering for his attention, and you could see the look of envy on the other passengers' faces, because whenever they came close, the tortoises would retreat, either away from the fence or back into the safety of their shells. Not so with Trevor – the tortoise whisperer!

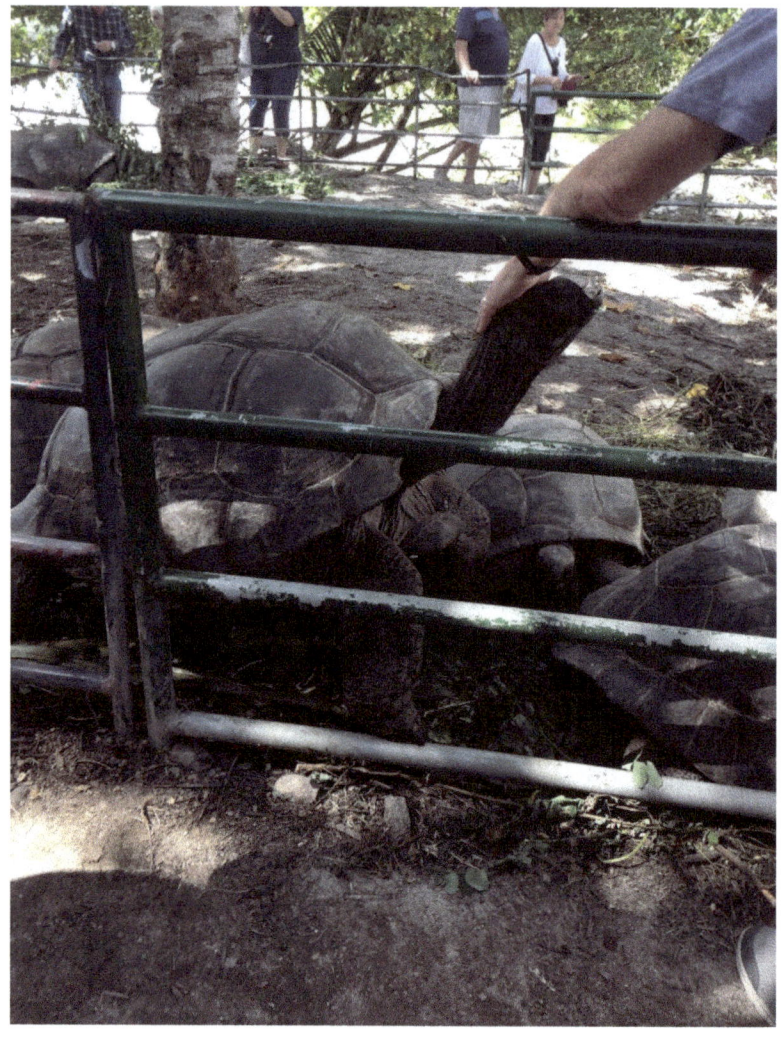

Trevor petting the tortoises - they couldn't get enough of him!

We then got back onto our respective buses, and whilst we were driving, there was really no need to speak and, if really necessary, I was able to manage the few words I needed without seeming rude.

The next shore trip however was Zanzibar, and this was a different story altogether. Trevor and I were on totally different tours, although we did see a lot of the same places. This is the town where Freddie Mercury (from the famous group 'Queen') was born. I had never been here before and was shocked and deeply moved by the dreadful history of slavery that had occurred here. It appalled me that so much poverty still prevailed. This ancient, exotic, primitive island seemed to be in a time warp that saw everything – and everyone – stuck in the 19th century.

As we were assembling outside, ready to go into the Princess Lounge prior to disembarking the ship, I realised I'd left my cruise card in the cabin. I wouldn't be able to get off the ship if I didn't have this, because the ship's security staff scan it every time you go on or off the ship. This is how they know who is on board and who hasn't yet returned.

When I got back and wanted to register as the tour escort (by showing my ticket that said I was the escort – I personally couldn't say it at this stage), they said they had no more tour escort tickets, so they just gave me a passenger ticket. 'Someone' was looking after me, because this saved me from having to verbalise the way tour escorts are supposed to do. I could sit there just like any other passenger.

Later when we were on our buses, the tour guide asked who the escort was and I just put up my hand, let him know my name and left it at that – it was all I could manage to say.

Just before the tour ended, we all went to quite a grand hotel where we had a choice of drink. We were seated at various-sized tables and I was with a couple about my age. We were looking over the beautiful water, watching the sailing boats and small waves lapping the shoreline. I knew that my ability to communicate and verbalise was getting more difficult and I tried to avoid eye contact because I didn't want to get into any conversation. However, the man sitting opposite me decided he would make some small talk.

My mind could not bring forth what I wanted to say. I knew exactly what he was saying to me. I knew exactly how I would have normally responded, and I could hear my response inside my head, but that bit in my brain that actually puts these two things together, so they happen one after the other, was not functioning. I had no words.

He just looked at me, obviously waiting for me to respond. After all, it wasn't rocket science we were discussing, although it well could have been, given my inability to relate with him on the same level.

I felt really embarrassed and tried to cover this by saying: 'Sorry, but I have a speech impediment.'

Looking back, I find it hard to comprehend how I was able to manage to say these relatively big words and couldn't get out some simple small talk. Maybe it was because I'd had a bit of time to push the words out and, deep down, I knew this would work to shut down any further interaction, which it did.

His response was one that still haunts me and one I'll never forget. He literally turned his back to me and in that moment I understood how people who can't communicate properly get treated. I understood the loneliness and isolation they must feel. It wasn't his fault, really. A lot of people don't know how to communicate with people when it is so one-sided. They often mistake lack of ability to communicate with lack of intelligence and for the most part, people just feel inadequate themselves in this situation.

I was just glad he didn't try to talk more slowly, more condescendingly and louder as so many people often do.

A voice inside me was saying: 'This isn't really me. I'm usually very articulate. I really don't have a speech impediment – it's just something to say to excuse my problem. Please don't shut me out. Please talk to me even though I can't talk back to you. Please don't exclude me.'

When we returned to the ship, I told Trevor that I wouldn't be doing any more shore tours but that I really wanted him to go, because I didn't want him to miss out on these wonderful experiences and opportunities that might never come around again. Besides, we were going to be going to Richards Bay in a few days' time and there would be wonderful safaris that he could experience. I didn't want him to miss out on anything because of me. After all, he could take photos and tell me everything that he saw and did, and I could share it that way.

Reluctantly he agreed.

Secretly, I knew things weren't improving for me, and with him gone on a shore tour, he would be away and I could hide it from him a little longer. Also, I wouldn't have to watch him looking at me, when he thought I wasn't looking, with grave concern written all over his face.

On February 13 we were anchored out of *Nosy Be* (pronounced Nosey Bay) in Madagascar and because it was really hot and we'd been there before, we decided to give it a miss. Unfortunately for the passengers who hadn't ever been there, the ship was declined entry by the port authorities due to the coronavirus, so we all missed out.

At this stage there had been a big problem on the Diamond Princess, which at that time was in Japan. There were confirmed cases on board of passengers who had coronavirus. They had been confined to their staterooms and extra precautions were also being taken so as not to spread the virus.

We had no idea at this stage of the impact this virus would have on people's health, their livelihood, as well as the global economy and the number of lives that would be lost as a result.

Being really conscious of the measures the ships take whenever there is something potentially contagious on board, we thought the Diamond Princess would have things in hand soon. Even **they** didn't know the magnitude of what they were dealing with.

Trevor and I even joked a bit about it all, with him saying: 'Imagine being confined to a room with no break from each other for a few weeks. I love you dearly, but I think I'd go crazy!'

During this period, where I'd been keeping to myself more, so as not to bring attention to my problem, Trevor did so much to try to support me. I knew he was really worried, even though he didn't say as much to me. One of the things he suggested that he thought might be helpful, to exercise and stimulate my brain a bit, was that we go and have a game of Scrabble.

For those of you who don't know me, Scrabble is my love. I just love the challenge of making words and getting big scores as well. Okay ... let's be honest... I love to win! I think I get this from my parents. Although Dutch, they played Scrabble (in English) for many, many years and they had a running tally of who won games. They were pretty much neck and neck at the time of their last game together and I think I'm just doing my bit to honour this family tradition.

So, I thought this was a great idea. However, my brain seemed to have other ideas. I found it very difficult to make complex words and I also had problems making more than two words at any time. I used to love it when I could make lots of words in one go (Scrabble players will know what I'm talking about).

When we had another game, Trevor suggested that I score. I agreed, but I couldn't switch from making words to counting scores, let alone writing them down. I was so grateful that he didn't make a big deal of it – he just took over the scoring.

It's difficult to describe the feeling I had in my head. I didn't experience any pain. I didn't feel any discomfort. I just had this sensation of it all just being too much. It felt like I was totally overwhelmed. I was overloading my thinking. It was like eye strain of my brain! If anything, I felt like my brain wasn't big enough to contain everything and that it was all too compressed, and I couldn't separate my individual thoughts or feelings. Thankfully, this feeling wasn't prolonged. As soon as there wasn't any pressure to think or act put on me in any way, everything was okay ...

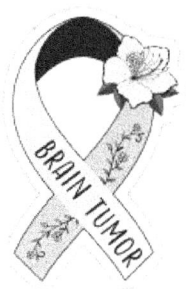

*Love is the happiness
Found in the realisation
That each moment you have
Is yours to appreciate.*

*Love is that rare commodity
That is never ending.*

*The more you give,
The more you have to give.*

CHAPTER 7

February 14 – Valentine's Day

Fairytales have a lot to answer for. They are responsible for the yearnings, the fantasies and the unreal expectations of women today. We're led to believe that we're equal and that we're independent, but this is not the case.

When it comes to romance, we're slaves to unreal expectations.

We wait for our handsome prince, our knight in shining armour. Then we wait for that magic moment ... the moment when their eyes meet ours, when their lips meet ours in that wonderful first kiss... that moment when the rest of the world stands still, and nothing exists but each other... the moment we know that our own fairytale is coming true and we're going to live happily ever after.

It was like that when I met Trevor. I thought I'd hit the jackpot. Not only had I met the man of my dreams, I had also met the man who could fulfill all my romantic fantasies.

You see, Trevor is a singer and when he sings to me, I melt. He has the voice of an angel. Actually, that's not really true ...

because when he sings to me, it doesn't really inspire me to be good (if you know what I mean).

But we're married and have been for 17 years now, so now romance often takes a back seat to life.

In reality, up until the last few years, we had actually spent more time apart than we did together.

I used to wonder what the expression 'absence makes the heart grow fonder' was really all about. I realise now that it's because when you're apart and you think about each other, you don't think dinner, dishes, dogs, dirty laundry, dusting and all those demoralising 'D' words that can **destroy** romance.

Instead, you're thinking love and you're reliving, recreating and romanticising it.

Romance is that vital ingredient that determines whether the relationship sizzles or fizzles and we have always wanted it to sizzle. We knew that this did not just happen automatically and as a result, we had to take steps to ensure it did. This is still the case now that we spend most of our time together, either on the farm or cruising.

Like most guys though, Trevor isn't really one for all the materialistic, showy romantic gestures. In fact, he doesn't get what all the fuss is about. He doesn't want to give a present or do something sweet just because it's expected of him. However, with my upbringing in the realm of fantasy and romance, I have often felt short-changed in this department.

Valentine's Day several years ago now, was no exception, except that Trevor wasn't even home. He was having a romantic time on the high seas (romantic, in the sailor/adventurer sense, that is).

I was home, all alone!

And to compound it, we weren't even in the same time zone. He was in my yesterday and I was in his tomorrow.

He arrived home three days later, and although Valentine's Day wasn't mentioned as such, he was home and so was the promise of romance ... after we cooked tea, emptied his suitcase, washed and ironed his clothes, fed and watered the animals and attended to what needed to be attended to... you know how it is ... life gets in the way. You talk about events rather than your dreams and you live a realistic life rather that a life realised.

Well, whilst feeding the animals, Trevor was really concerned about some strange markings on the ground in one of our paddocks and he wanted to get my opinion. A few years ago, we'd had three huge, perfectly symmetrical shapes on our top paddock that looked like crop circles, which we could never explain.

He walked hand in hand with me and I looked and looked some more thinking all the while how strange it was. I hadn't even noticed it prior to this, despite feeding Jericho, our stallion, for the past few weeks, right near that very spot.

There in front of me was a very strange pattern of dead grass, but it wasn't in a circular shape like the strange ones we'd seen before. Also, it was nowhere near as big. I couldn't make it out and Trevor said: 'Have a closer look.'

And then I saw it!

A few weeks earlier, Trevor had been poisoning weeds with Roundup along the fence lines and obviously he'd gotten a bit carried away because there, written in dead grass, was a big heart with an arrow going through it and the words 'T loves M'.

He had decided to do something really special for me, something no one has ever done for me and probably never will again. That's right, girls! For Valentine's Day I got dead grass!

'Happy Valentine's Day' he cooed in my ear.

So as far as I'm concerned now, you can keep your perfect red roses. You can keep your fancy dinners. You can keep your chocolates. I'd rather have dead grass any day!

Since that Valentine's Day, we have always made a point of doing something special, with lots of forethought for each other.

This year we were both on a cruise and weeks before we left, I'd bought Trevor a really special card that was a reminder of when we'd first met.

I remember that first fateful meeting – hard to believe it was 17 years ago. Trevor had said to his friend, Michael: 'I don't think I'll ever find anyone I could be with for the rest of my life. In fact, I doubt if someone like that could even exist.'

That same day, 17 years ago, although I didn't voice it, I was also contemplating relationships and had come to the conclusion that marriage and long-term commitment was probably a thing in my past. I was happy and content with the thought of being single. It wasn't that I didn't like men. I really enjoyed male company, but I felt my life was really quite full and complete as it was.

So, the reality was that neither of us believed anything was missing in our lives, nor were we looking for a partner in life. This is usually when Cupid steps in and shoots his arrow. It's interesting that sometimes you don't know how empty things really are, until you experience the magic of true love and fulfilment.

So, when neither of us was looking, we found each other and since then there has been nobody else for either of us.

This was what I wanted to convey in my card. I had written a little note inside the card prior to leaving home but had been called away and hadn't had time to finish it. So, on the morning of Valentine's Day, whilst Trevor was in the shower, I finished writing on the card. It is quite obvious (now) by the fact that I repeated myself, and the fact that my writing had changed, that I was really having problems and that these were now extending to my written expression.

There was also a noticeable reduction in the strength in my right hand. At the time, I wasn't aware of the degree these things had changed, but later Trevor pointed out to me that this had been a real defining moment for him because the signs were now so clearly visible.

Again, Trevor said nothing to me, but I know he did have some conversations with Hans and Rowena, and they talked about the way my condition was progressing – and not for the better.

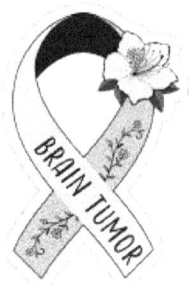

You must trust that the Universe

Will give you all you need.

Be patient and trusting

For all will come to pass as it must.

Life's teardrops are but splashes on the

whirlpool of life.

CHAPTER 8

Saturday, February 15

I had noticed that now my body was getting a little bit weaker, and I had even had a few issues with bladder control. At one stage I couldn't get my shorts off quickly enough and I wet myself all over them. This was really embarrassing for me and I made a point of going to the toilet more often so that I wouldn't be caught short, so to speak. This again was tied up with my right-side muscle weakness.

Then on February 15, after a restless night where I'd had trouble getting comfortable, I noticed that I had lost the strength on my right side. I was sleeping on the top bunk in our cabin and could hardly raise myself up to sitting position.

'How on earth am I going to get myself down from here?' I said to myself.

And then the thoughts started to stockpile.

'Oh my God! I'm having a stroke. But how can that be? I'm only 63, and I'm fit and healthy.'

There was nothing for it but to finally admit there was something really wrong, and I had to talk to Trevor about it.

Between sobs, which exacerbated my already incoherent speech, I told him very briefly what I suspected. He helped me to the bottom end of the bed and down the ladder. Then he sat me down in the chair opposite him. He was very quiet as he let me talk. He held me in his arms, transferring to me, the emotional strength I was lacking in that moment.

As it turned out, I think he had been waiting for me to say it was time to get some expert medical help so we could find out what was really wrong with me.

He took charge immediately and this was such a relief to me. Normally I like to be very much in control, especially with regards to my life and decisions that concern me. Normally I don't like anyone just taking over, especially without asking me first. But this was no normal situation, and I was caught up in this rollercoaster where I was losing control over my most basic bodily functions.

I wanted him to be there and take over for me, because I could no longer do it. I couldn't trust that my body wouldn't fail me, and I had lost the capacity to think through things and make rational decisions.

In, and from that moment, Trevor became my lifeline whilst I battled against the turbulent sea of confusion and aphasia. I felt like a swimmer caught in an undertow, drowning in my fears and, just like that swimmer, I could fight it no longer.

Trevor was my lifesaver. I felt so safe in his arms, and I knew without a doubt that he would move Heaven and Earth to get me the best care he possibly could.

He sprang into action immediately. He made a phone call to the medical centre and said he'd be down shortly because he needed to talk to them. He told me he wanted to talk to them by himself so he could explain what had been happening over the past week or so and give them a thorough background.

He was really worried about me being alone, so he said he was going to drop me off at Hans and Rowena's cabin, while he went to the medical centre aboard the ship.

I was a mess. I had so many different thoughts flit through my head. Thoughts about how helpless I was feeling; thoughts about my own mortality, and worse still, thoughts about a future that I didn't want, one where I couldn't walk or talk.

My world as I knew it, was crumbling around me and I felt vulnerable, not knowing what was going to become of the 'me' I'd gotten used to being. I had always been such a strong person, so dependable and here I was, scared, vulnerable and dependent. I didn't want this, but I was now on a trajectory that I was unable to escape from. I was along for the ride whether I liked it or not.

I was also really concerned about the implications of my not being well. After all, Trevor still had shows to do.

I felt I was letting everybody down.

What would the cruise director have to say about this?

Would she be angry that I'd put her in a predicament where she'd have to organise other acts at short notice? It was usually us who offered our extra shows, workshops and talks at short notice and pulled a rabbit out of the proverbial hat.

Would we ever be invited back on after this fiasco?

And the cost ... oh my God, the cost!

Not only would we have to pay all the on-board hospital bills (which could run into thousands of dollars) up front, what if the travel insurance we had wouldn't cover it?

If I thought I couldn't think straight before, now I was overwhelmed with my thoughts and as far as I believed at that time, none of them had a good outcome.

The drowning feeling was there again as I gave into these thoughts and found myself gasping for breath. It was such a relief and comfort to me when I got to Hans and Rowena's room, knowing they were there to support me, no matter what, and on my terms. There was no judgment from them; no 'you should have gone to the doctor earlier' – only unconditional love.

They let me cry and made soothing noises as I sat between them both, and their comforting embrace was an elixir to my fears and had a wonderful, calming influence upon me.

Within 30 minutes, Trevor came back and said he'd spoken to the doctor. He told me I was to go down to the medical centre so they could examine me. I know Trevor was so glad he could do this for me. I think he really needed to do something. He needed to feel useful. I know he was scared as well, but at this stage, when we had no answers, he was just glad he could be instrumental in getting me to where I needed to go on the path to getting some answers.

As he said to me so many times over the following weeks: 'Worry is just a down payment on fear.'– *James Bond*.

Thank goodness there was no one around to see this emotional, tear-streaked, wreck of a woman, me, being escorted down to level four medical centre.

The nurse on duty immediately took my vital signs. Given my level of emotional distress, my blood pressure was sky high. This of course led them to believe I was indeed having a stroke.

I was admitted and examined more thoroughly by another nurse and two doctors and was monitored from that moment on.

Initially there was talk about getting me airlifted to the nearest land hospital via helicopter. Fortunately, my vital signs had stabilised, and the second doctor had some doubts about the diagnosis because I still had quite a bit of strength in my right leg, despite the fact my right arm was very weak, and I had a distinctive droop to the right side of my mouth.

The doctors said they wished I had come earlier because then they might have been able to treat me more appropriately, and at an earlier stage.

I know for a fact though, I would have refused any treatment that acted as a blood thinner prior to a brain scan. The reason for this was that my ex-husband had had a stroke when he was 50 (a number of years after our divorce), and he is a shadow of his former self. He is now severely disabled, due to marked brain damage caused by another, subsequent, huge bleed in his brain. Also, I had known other people who'd had massive bleeds due to the wrong medication.

As it turned out, it was fate that we did what we did and decided to wait. So, by luck or good judgment, we had indeed made the right decision.

I was admitted to the on-board hospital and the staff continued to monitor me.

They asked Trevor to bring up some toiletries and anything else I might need because, as far as they were concerned, I was there to stay, at least until we reached our next port of call. This certainly wasn't in my plan. I thought I'd be able to sort a few things out and come back, but they wouldn't have a bar of this. They also asked Trevor to give them our travel insurance details so they could start to sort out the process of being paid.

This daunting task of sorting out our belongings in preparation for leaving the ship fell on Rowena's shoulders. She had kindly volunteered to do it, not really knowing what she was getting herself into. She went down to the cabin with Trevor, and they were shocked at the disarray of all my belongings in the cabin. On the surface everything looked okay, but when they opened cupboards and drawers, it was a totally different picture.

I am usually very organised. I like everything in its place and on board I have a system so I know exactly where things are, where I can access anything and everything really easily and, when it comes to packing at the end of a cruise, I can do so very quickly. In fact, I get annoyed when things get moved and when Trevor puts his things in 'my place'.

Because Trevor and I do a variety of shows on board, we need to bring a lot of luggage. I also insist on bringing our fabulous healthy shakes and nutritional supplements with us as well when we travel.

They both said it was an absolute nightmare! Trevor couldn't believe his eyes because things were everywhere. I've often said to Trevor that 'the state you keep your belongings in, is a true indicator of where your mind is at' – and when he saw the mess in front of him, he started to fathom and understand the level of disarray my mind must be in.

There was no order to anything. Trevor usually doesn't venture into my storage space, but he had to in this case. He couldn't make head nor tail of it. He told me later that it had taken him most of the night to pack for us both and in the end, he'd just thrown things in suitcases as best he could, figuring he could sort it all out later.

The amazing thing though, was that Trevor and Rowena told me this afterwards. It was something I wasn't even aware of, and even now, given how pedantic I can be, I still find it unbelievable.

I am so sorry they had to go through this and do this for me, but I suppose, looking on the bright side now, it certainly gave them something else to focus on.

I'm glad they didn't tell me at the time because I would have been really embarrassed about it and I would have insisted that I personally go down to sort it out. After all, I was just lying there doing nothing much.

The worst of it though, they said, was trying to find our Cover-More Travel Insurance details and card. I was the one who always organised a yearly cover for us both. We do it yearly because this is the most economical way to do it and also, we then know we are covered for the whole year. I put a note in my diary and always get the best rates as well, doing it when Flight Centre has its annual yearly promotional sale. I usually give Trevor a card and I also keep one in my purse, but I had omitted to do it on this occasion. I really never expected we would have to use it.

Naturally, Trevor thought the card would be in my purse, but it wasn't. Fortunately, he did have a card from the previous year and knew that I had renewed it a few months prior, in October last year, so he figured if he asked me, I would just be able to tell him where it was, which I thought I did: 'It's in the room,' I said.

So, Trevor and Rowena went back and looked in the top drawer, where I usually keep important things, but it wasn't there. They then looked, and looked, and looked and looked and then looked some more, but alas! It was nowhere to be seen. They then went back to the medical centre to ask me: 'Where in the room is it?'

I told them it was in the computer, so they searched for a file named Cover-More Travel Insurance. Again, they came back to me, trying to hide their frustration, saying: 'It's not there.'
I then said: 'It is. It's in an email from Flight Centre.'
They were then able to start the process of putting in the insurance claim.

This was a really good example of how my brain was working (or should I say, not working). I can now understand the frustration they must have felt. It was such a simple thing. I had access to all the bits of information, but I couldn't get my brain to put the pieces of information together in a way that was logical. Also, everything I was saying in dribs and drabs seemed quite understandable and rational to me at the time.

It was like being asked to retrieve a file from a filing cabinet (my brain) where each of the files (information) has been mixed up with everything else and there is no alphabet or other system to help you instantly put your hands onto what it is you're looking for.

Never once did they lash out at me though. I think they knew I was trying my best and that this was the best I could do at the time.

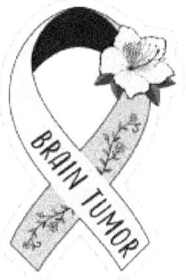

Be grateful for each
And every obstacle in your life
For it provides another opportunity
To grow and define
The true being
Of 'who' you are

CHAPTER 9

Monday, February 17

On the early morning of February 17, we should have been on a tour, excitedly venturing out in the wilderness, enjoying the wonders of nature that only Africa can provide.

Instead, we were venturing into our own wilderness, unsure of the outcome and very unsure of what this day would bring.

All the arrangements had been finalised for an ambulance to transfer me from the Sun Princess to just outside the wharf area where I would be transferred by another ambulance, attached to Richards Bay Hospital to be taken there for an MRI scan of my brain. The reason for two ambulances was that one ambulance is authorised by the port authorities and the other is attached to the hospital ambulance service. The second one has no derestriction in the port area and the first ambulance is not able to go out of this area in case they are called to another medical emergency.

At first the medical centre staff on board were not sure which hospital they would send me to, but on a recommendation from a very good friend of Trevor's daughter, Bronwyn, it was suggested I be taken to Netcare, The Bay Hospital.

This ended up being another one of those decisions, that initially didn't seem particularly important, but in the end proved to be another of the miracles we encountered.

Rowena and Hans had booked a safari and they were going out with a small group of people. This had been privately booked and they were due to return to the ship at 4.30pm just prior to it sailing for Cape Town. We had assured them we would let them know if we needed them, but for now, they were on a holiday and we didn't want what was happening to me to interfere with their plans. Besides, Trevor and I had been told to leave all our belongings on board because the likelihood was, that I had had a stroke, and I would be able to come back on board and fly home, as was planned, when we got to Cape Town.

They said to each other: 'So typical of us. Over-reacting as usual. It's nowhere near as bad as we thought.'

So, after coming to the medical centre quite early that morning to say farewell for now, Hans, Rowena, Trevor and I arranged to catch up later that evening so we could hear about their wonderful adventures, and they could hear about our medical adventure. We were so glad they didn't change their plans, regardless of what happened in their absence.

Getting off the ship was pretty awful for me. I was sitting in a wheelchair and Trevor, security staff, a nurse, as well as a few deck hands were with me. The deck hands helped manoeuvre me (in the wheelchair) down the ramp.

I was aware of a number of people who had gathered to see me being taken off the ship. I knew there would be rumours and one of them was that I had coronavirus (we weren't calling it COVID-19 at that stage). It is human curiosity to have a sticky beak and I was well aware of this, but this made me feel really exposed and vulnerable, and again my emotions took flight and I found myself getting really upset, crying and making matters much worse, to the point of becoming totally unintelligible.

In the first ambulance the nurse gave a brief handover. They took my blood pressure and other vital signs. Then we were driven a kilometre or so to the next ambulance. They were given a quick handover and then I was transferred into the back.

There were two ambulance officers – Angelique, who was reassuring me as she got busy attaching their monitor equipment on me, and her co-worker, who was bombarding me with questions to try and get a history, chain of events and so on right from the get-go.

Trevor was with me in the back of the first ambulance, but he was not allowed to accompany me there in the second ambulance. For a start, there wasn't any room for him, and he was asked to sit up front with Angelique, who was driving. There was a partition between the back and front so he couldn't hear what was going on in the back.

Meanwhile, I was in the back with the other ambulance attendant, who continued to bombard me with questions, even though it was obvious I was having difficulty answering, not for lack of trying. These were questions that had already been asked and answered (maybe not to her specifically, but she had a copy of all the details).

I got really frustrated because there was no way I could communicate with her and I actually thought she lacked a lot of empathy and compassion. After all, it was pretty obvious that I couldn't speak; and it was pretty obvious that I was being taken to hospital for a brain scan because of this; and it was pretty obvious that this was not normal for me...

Trevor couldn't hear me, even though I could hear him, and I couldn't understand why he wasn't responding to some of my garbled muffles of distress as I tried to get his attention. I wanted him to speak to Zama on my behalf, but he was just chatting with Angelique, oblivious to what I was going through. What I didn't realise, and am eternally grateful for now, is that Angelique, by engaging him in normal conversation, was able to get a lot more information, including background, recent events, why we were in Richards Bay and Trevor was able to chat with her in a relaxed manner while she also gave him a mini tour of the environs from the port to the hospital.

In hindsight, although I still believe strongly that the ambulance attendee with me could have handled the situation so much better with a little bit of reassurance, a little bit of calm and an explanation to me of where we were going, how long it would take and what she was doing with me, I must accept some responsibility for overreacting and making things worse.

I was just so relieved when we finally got to the hospital and, once again, I had Trevor by my side. I realised at this stage how dependent I'd become on him. He was the person who understood me and spoke for me and made me feel safe.

The ambulance crew exchanged information with the hospital staff when we arrived, and I was put into a wheelchair and taken down the hall where we waited just outside the MRI department. After about 15 minutes, I was wheeled in for the

MRI scan of my brain. Trevor sat on a seat just outside and waited, and waited, and waited. It took about 90 minutes.

The technicians explained to me that it might be a bit uncomfortable because I would be lying on a table that would slide into the machine. They said there would be a lot of loud, clanging type noises and also that it might be a scary experience, particularly if I suffered from claustrophobia. They stressed though, the most important thing was I had to keep my head very still the entire time.

I probably knew all of this before, but again, never did I think I would have to go through it myself.

I am very claustrophobic – I even hate being in a confined lift and I don't do underground roads or tunnels or caves for that very reason.

They gave me a buzzer and said if I really couldn't cope, I was to press this or just raise my hand and they would take me out of the machine.

However, when you have no choice and the need far outweighs the fear, you do whatever is necessary. I also knew that no matter how difficult I found it, if I asked for a break, I would not have the strength to be put back into the machine.

So, in I went, and the journey of discovery began.

I decided to close my eyes and keep them closed throughout the entire procedure.

Well, the machine was everything they said and more, but I felt a calm come over me. I felt this amazing strength that you can only get from within. I relaxed into it, breathed deeply and saw in my mind the people I love and the experiences I have had and am so grateful for. This is what got me through it.

The technician brought me out after about an hour and then said she needed to get a few more pictures. She didn't tell me more than this. I already knew things weren't right – that there was something wrong and I knew she really had to pinpoint exactly what it was and that this could be tricky. I rationalised it, thinking I must have moved or that she just needed to get some clearer pictures. After all, I didn't see that look on her face that said ... 'Oh my God!' so I didn't worry too much. We were in a different country and maybe procedures were different here.

This time it was a little harder to get into the groove, but I thought: 'This is really important. They have obviously found something and need some more pictures to be sure. I just need to focus and to be calm.'

Again, this amazing strength came out of nowhere.

I knew they'd found something, but we had to wait until the technicians finished their analysis and then passed on their findings to the emergency department doctor.

The doctor wasn't available right away, but the nurse looking after me said to Trevor: 'We're going to be keeping her in.'

At this stage he realised they'd found something serious, but he didn't know exactly what – maybe another stroke?

We would not be returning to the ship and sailing to the next few ports, but hopefully we'd still be flying home as planned.

So as a result, Trevor had to go back and get our luggage from the ship.

The only problem was that this had all been locked up in the medical centre, which of course was closed when he got there. He did manage to track down the cruise director and the medical doctor and relayed what he knew at this stage (which was very little). He was able to retrieve the luggage, which he then had to get off the ship (all 80 kilograms of it).

The people at Princess Cruises were wonderful. The port agent, Norman, had been notified and he, in collaboration with Princess Cruises, organised and made arrangements for Trevor to stay at the Indaba Lodge, with all meals included, as well as transport to and from the hospital. They arranged transport immediately to drop him back to the hospital so that he could be with me and arranged for his luggage to go to the Indaba Lodge. I don't think they realised how very much this meant to us ... and this was just the beginning of all their support.

Being in a strange country, Trevor realised he would need a local SIM card he could use in South Africa. The driver stopped at a local convenience store and got him a card with the equivalent of $AU20 on it to temporarily tide him over. The following day, Trevor was able to exchange some Australian dollars for some African rand and repay the driver.

It was really difficult for Trevor to contact Hans and Rowena to let them know what had happened. However, he was able to leave a message on their cabin phone saying we were staying in Richards Bay. He told them I was being admitted because they'd found something that warranted it. Naturally, Trevor assumed it was another stroke, so that was basically the message he left.

Hans and Rowena had no way to contact us directly, and I subsequently learned that they phoned the hospital just prior to the ship departing. The woman to whom they spoke did not appear to understand what they were saying and told Hans that Trevor had left the hospital and then she terminated the call. He had only left temporarily to go back to the ship to pick up our luggage and was on his way back, but the impression she'd left them with was that Trevor had just abandoned me. They thought this was very unlikely, but they had no way of getting any further information. He wasn't on the ship, so where was he?

When Trevor got back to the hospital, he came in to see me in the emergency department (bed five) and relayed what had happened on the ship. We thought it would probably just be a few days that I'd be in hospital. They would stabilise me and then we would both fly home, as planned.

The emergency department doctor was free soon after Trevor got back, and he asked Trevor if he would mind coming with him so he could talk to him in private.

This was a strange situation for me. From being so distressed earlier on, I was now very, very calm. I didn't even mind that Trevor left and talked to the doctor without me. Normally I would have said: 'If it's got to do with me, I want in on the conversation.'

I'm so glad I didn't say this though, because what they found was horrific.

After the doctor showed Trevor the pictures of the brain scan, he said: 'Now you tell her!'

I don't know where Trevor found the strength to do this. I think it's because we've never had any secrets and he knows me so well and knew I would want to know.

He sat opposite me as I sat on the side of the bed. He held my hand and, looking me straight in the eye, he said: 'Maya, it's really bad. They've found a really big tumour on your brain.'

I remember feeling shocked because I really hadn't expected this. I didn't know what to say as the reality of what he'd just said started to sink in.

I remembered people I'd known of in the past who'd died a horrific death soon after being diagnosed with a brain tumour, so I was under no illusion about how bad things potentially could be.

Because I had had no symptoms prior to the cruise, and now the tumour was huge (the size of a tennis ball, they said), plus the symptoms were so markedly obvious and getting worse every day, I felt that, if I did survive, things would get much worse and very quickly. Eventually I would be a mere shadow of myself.

The first thing that came into my mind was that I was likely to die ... and soon.

I had to let Trevor know that I wasn't scared for me and that I was ready to die if it came to that. I told him I wasn't afraid to die.

To this he said: 'That may be so, but I don't want to lose you and we will fight it in whatever way we can, together as we've always done.'

So now we were on this road together, not knowing how long we would share the journey and not knowing where it would end for us.

I'm so glad it was Trevor who told me about the diagnosis and not the doctor. It was such a personal thing, and hearing this from a stranger was not what I wanted, no matter how sympathetic or empathic he might have said it. Also, I don't think I would have reacted with such grace and clarity as I did when Trevor told me. I think that for Trevor, it was one of the most difficult things he ever had to do and for that I felt such gratitude that he told me gently, but honestly.

We never know how we will react when faced with our own mortality and it really surprised me that I was so calm about it.

I truly had no fear whatsoever. I hoped it would be quick and painless and I had more concern for those I would leave behind than for myself. I have always had a strong belief in the afterlife and was not afraid to transition to this.

As soon as possible, Trevor sent a text to Hans and Rowena to let them know the results of the MRI. He didn't know how to tell them, so he just wrote: 'There's nothing for it but to tell you bluntly. Maya has a brain tumour. It's the size of a tennis ball.'

They sent him back a text, saying they'd received his message.

They were dumbstruck. They didn't text this but told me later that it made them feel so sorry for us, knowing what our future was likely to look like. They were also sad that they were potentially going to lose me within the next few months. They battled with so many confusing emotions ... mostly this awful feeling of helplessness (probably much like Trevor).

Hans had worked in the neurology ward and had extensive experience (albeit not personally) of what this diagnosis could mean. However, this time it was different, because this time it was me, his sister, and that made it very personal.

They went down to see the doctors and nurses in the ship's medical centre and updated them with the latest information. They were shocked as to the diagnosis – especially as there were no warning signs (not even a headache) and Francois, the senior doctor asked if they would keep him updated as to my progress, which they continued to do.

Hans and Rowena tried to phone us in the ICU, not realising I wasn't there yet and wouldn't be admitted there for 30 hours. They were quite frustrated with the lack of communication initially, but this is what happens when a crisis you're not expecting hits you or your loved ones on land, and you are on a ship in the Indian Ocean. You want all the answers **now** and sometimes there just aren't any there and then.

A lot of things needed to play out first and a lot of procedures needed to be done following the initial diagnosis that even we weren't aware of.

Between themselves, Hans and Rowena talked about different options and how they could help. They relayed these to Trevor over the next few days and told him that rather than go on a tour in Durban, they would take the trip to see us both when they got to Durban (this was a 2.5 hour trip by car).

They realised it was up to us to decide what we'd like from them, but they wanted to table what they were prepared to do so we could give it some serious consideration. They were both prepared to give up their cabin to us if I was unable to fly home and they in turn would catch a plane home, thereby cutting their holiday short. They were also prepared for Rowena, as a nurse, to fly home with me if I was deemed stable enough. They were also open to staying in Richards Bay to support us. They knew all this would be dependent on medical advice and the ship captain's discretion.

We were so surprised by their level of thoughtfulness and generosity towards us. I know we're family but it's not usually until anyone is really put to the test that you realise their true value and see what they're really made of. They were even talking about postponing the next world cruise they had planned. They had only just booked it and it was scheduled to leave in May 2020 (a few months' time). I remember when they were telling us about it. They were both really excited and told us about the specific ports it would stop at (ones the world cruise doesn't usually do). We could feel this excitement and were so thrilled for them.

Trevor and I decided to wait and see how things progressed. I knew full well that I didn't want them to cut their holiday short on any account, nor did I want them to miss out on any future holidays, but I didn't argue at that time.

We were really surprised when not long after Trevor told me my diagnosis, Angelique, the ambulance driver came into my room in the emergency department. She had been curious about the outcome of the MRI and, although she'd been relieved when she found out it wasn't a stroke, this relief was short-lived when she discovered I had a tumour.

Enjoying the learning side of everything in this fascinating job as an ambulance officer, she felt a bit torn between her medical fascination with the tumour and its presenting symptoms, and the fear she felt for me as a person now she'd gotten to know us both a bit. She wondered to herself: 'If I got this news, what would I want? What would comfort me? Ah, I know. Chocolate always does the trick.'

So, she went out and bought me a small bar of Cadbury milk chocolate, walked into my room and said how sorry she was to hear our sad news and placed this chocolate in my hands saying: 'I know it's not much, but I wanted to give you something of comfort and all I could think of was chocolate.'

I can't begin to tell you how touched I was by this small, but thoughtful action. This woman, who barely knew us, had taken time out of her day to come and see me and give me a gift – a gift that represented 'who' she was. I kept this bar of chocolate as a precious memento and reminder of the selflessness and kindness of others. When I finally did eat it, just prior to my discharge, I did so in her honour, fully mindful of the sensations it evoked on my palate and the positive emotions and gratitude I felt towards her.

That evening Dr. Krittish Timakia, the only neurosurgeon in that entire region, contacted Trevor and asked him to come to his rooms to discuss my condition, the prognosis and options for treatment.

One of the first things Trevor said to him was: 'Don't sugarcoat anything. I want to know all the facts and I want to know what I need to expect so I can be prepared.'

Be careful what you ask for ...

Trevor learned very early in the piece that Dr. Timakia is pedantic, precise, and honest about worst-case scenarios. But, thankfully, he was 'Heaven-sent' and extremely meticulous and dedicated.

He gave Trevor all the facts and then some more. He showed him my scans and discussed these. He showed him pictures (quite graphic ones) indicating everything that could go wrong in surgery, as well as complications post-surgery. He wanted him to really know how serious the situation was, so Trevor had the facts to face this head-on.

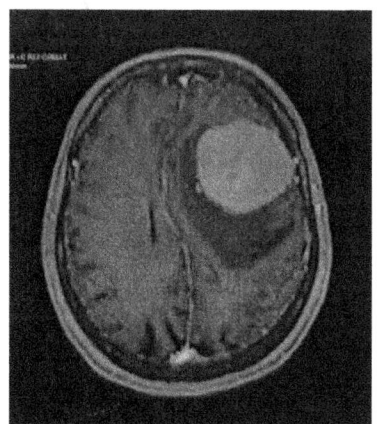

He wanted Trevor to understand there was a real urgency for medical intervention. In fact, Dr. Timakia was surprised I hadn't had a huge seizure already, one from which he said, I would have gone into a coma and not survived. He gave me a life expectancy of a few months (something Trevor didn't tell me until just recently).

When he showed Trevor the pictures of the MRI, these showed very clearly both the size of the tumour (tennis ball-sized), as well as its location and the way it was encroaching on the right hemisphere of my brain.

Dr. Timakia said one of the first things he would need to do was to decrease the swelling in my brain, so he started me on the appropriate medication to do this. He would also prescribe some medication to reduce the risk of seizures and he was going to transfer me to the ICU as soon as a suitable bed became available.

Trevor was with Dr. Timakia for about two hours and again I wasn't worried. I really was quite limited in my thoughts and was happy to lie there doing nothing. Usually, I'd be really impatient and want to read, do crosswords, do sudoku, hand sew, in fact anything to keep my hands or brain busy – but not anymore. Some part of me also instinctively realised that Trevor needed to talk with the specialist doctor on this level and have questions answered to his satisfaction.

Dr. Timakia said he would drive Trevor back to the Indaba Lodge (where the port agent had arranged for him to stay). This was such a kind gesture and so unexpected. It was 10pm by the time they left the hospital.

When Trevor came back to the emergency ward, he told me very briefly what Dr. Timakia had said. He knew, that although I would understand what he was telling me, I might be overwhelmed by too much information. My brain was indeed not able to process as much as it did before, and I was happy for this consideration.

He did say, however, that it didn't look good and that he had signed a Do Not Resuscitate (DNR) order on my behalf. I am grateful he did that and told him so. I know that living my life not in control of my basic physical functions and totally dependent upon others was not for me.

This had probably been the worst day in Trevor's life.

Within a short period, he'd had to leave the ship, go to the hospital, wait while I got a brain scan, go back to the ship, collect all our belongings, notify people of what was happening, see the pictures of my tumour, have to tell me, have to talk with the neurosurgeon and then try to process it all ...

I can't begin to comprehend the angst he went through and all the while being so loving and kind to me.

He said he needed a good night's sleep so was going to ask the doctor in the emergency department for some Valium to ensure he could do so. I was so pleased he did this because he hadn't had much sleep the night before and I knew he really needed that time out where he could let his brain absorb the unabsorbable.

Before he left, we decided that my tumour needed a name, so we called it 'Fred'. Having a separate entity meant that it was something outside of me and, although it was growing inside my head and really making itself known, it wasn't of me. By naming it and giving it its own identity made me feel less emotionally attached to it and would make it easier to isolate it and therefore make Fred **dead**. We didn't know how yet, but this was a really important thing for us both to do.

I found it so easy to visualise Fred, even though I hadn't seen the scan. I saw him as a large, hard ball pushing his way around inside my head. Being the bully he was, he figured he would have the upper hand. He was pretty ugly and wouldn't show his face, but that's the way of sneaky bullies. I visualised him as everything that had always stood in the way of me feeling good about myself and achieving all my dreams. I had always allowed people's opinions to count more than my own and I had always felt like I wasn't quite good enough (the way a lot of us feel from time to time). Having Fred where I could see him, sitting menacingly in my left peripheral vision, I thought: 'You're in my sights, mate. You're what's stopped me achieving things in my life and once I'm rid of you, I do not need to hide behind you and the excuses you represent anymore.'

Due to the location of my tumour, the effect on my brain was that my thinking was often removed from the harshness of reality. It was like the Universe and everyone in it had my back, no matter what. It was like I would be able to cope, no matter what was in store. I was in a place of true acceptance. I had full comprehension with none of the worry. I was actually quite happy and at peace, while at the same time, I had a very real understanding of what Trevor was going through and tried to support him as best I could. I needed him to know I was okay, because it was important to me that when he went home, to Indaba Lodge, he didn't worry needlessly about how I was feeling (on top of all his other very real concerns). I understood and wanted to free him to take this much-needed time out for himself and not rush back to me.

That night, before the Valium hit, Trevor contacted Bronwyn, his daughter in Canada.

He told her what had happened and naturally she was terribly shocked. As is her way, she just let him talk and then immediately said: 'How can we help?'

She offered to transfer money and said she would contact Kristy, my daughter and Steven, my son (presently living with Kristy).

Bronwyn and Trevor have always been really close, and it was such a blessing he was able to talk with her and just let his emotions out in a way he couldn't do with me. She was his release valve when he needed it most.

'Miracle in Richards Bay - Escape from the Vortex' by Maya Knight

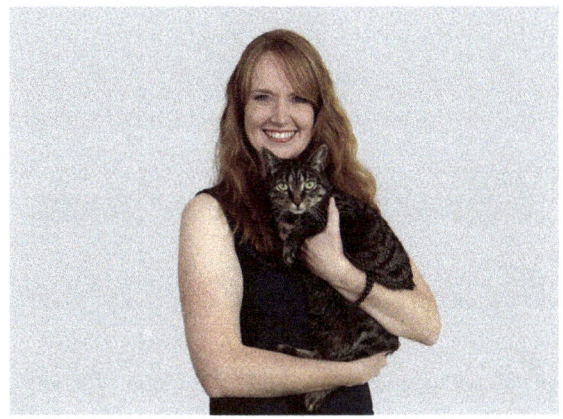

Bronwyn.

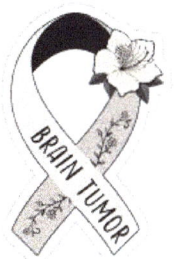

Be still in times of doubt.
Act steadfast in times of need.
Let your love keep you strong.
Let others sustain you.
Let your friends encourage you.
Let the hand of God touch you.

And never fear what lies ahead
For what lies within,
Expressed with love
Will see you through all turbulence
and hard times.

CHAPTER 10

Tuesday, February 18

Now that we knew what we were dealing with and had actually named it, there was so much to do...(or should I say, for Trevor to do).

Thankfully, he'd had a good night's sleep and was ready to face this new day all guns blazing, hoping for the best in what it would bring, knowing it really couldn't get much worse... or could it?

There was family to contact in Australia as well as in England and there was the unenviable task of sorting out the travel insurance. There was an eight-hour time difference between Australia and Richards Bay with Australia being ahead. There was a one-hour time difference between Richards Bay and England with Richards Bay being in front. There was a six-hour time difference between Toronto, Canada, where Trevor's daughter, Bronwyn lives and Richards Bay, with Toronto being behind. Also, due to daylight saving, there was an hour time difference between New South Wales, where Tristan, his son lives and Queensland, where Kristy and Steven, my children live, with Queensland being an hour behind. I don't know how Trevor kept track of it all, but he did. He also kept in regular contact with Princess Cruises in Los Angeles and they were nine hours behind. He didn't know if he was coming or going; in yesterday or today; and all the while, being conscious of the fact that people get really alarmed if the phone rings or they get alerted to emails at ungodly hours of the night. He certainly didn't want anyone alarmed any more than was necessary.

First things first, though! After he got back to Indaba Lodge the night before and got some semblance of unpacking done, he needed the type of logic and family support that only Tristan was really capable of providing, so he rang him.

Tristan is a pathologist working in the western suburbs of Sydney and he has the most incredibly retentive and analytical brain. He sees things that others often miss. Not only is he dedicated to his profession, he is also just as dedicated to his family (which of course extended to us).

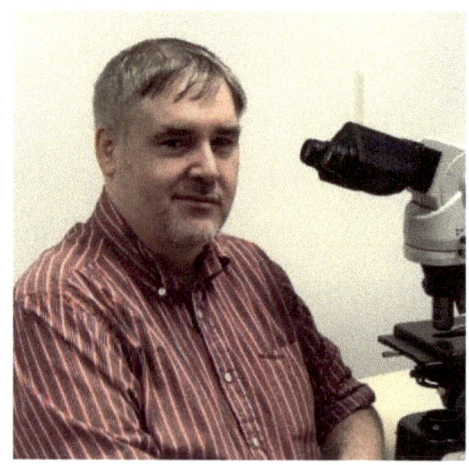

Tristan.

Tristan asked Trevor to ask Dr. Timakia to send all the scans to him so he could have a look at them (as long as Dr.Timakia was willing to do so). Trevor reassured him he would ask him as soon as he could, probably later in the morning when he could arrange it. We really didn't think he'd be amenable to this though.

Imagine our surprise (and Tristan's) when Dr.Timakia agreed to this without a moment's hesitation. We were gobsmacked that, unlike a lot of the specialists in Australia, Dr. Timakia did this and said he would be happy to send everything to Tristan and would also liaise with him and discuss my case with him in order to achieve the best outcome possible for me.

Tristan really was the perfect person in this scenario, being willing, able and extremely qualified to help us navigate our way through the medical maze in front of us.

We were once again reminded of Tristan's standing in the medical field, which sadly at times in the past, we had taken for granted. We were also amazed at Dr. Timakia's humility and quiet confidence. He didn't feel threatened in any way and this raised our opinions and confidence in him even more.

Trevor had also mentioned to Dr. Timakia that not only did Tristan have good connections with neurosurgeons, but

Bronwyn, his daughter in Canada, did as well. On hearing this, he also included Bronwyn on the list of people he CCd whenever he sent out emails with medical information about me.

Knowing all this and Dr. Timakia's willingness to work as a team, made us feel less isolated in this unfamiliar rainbow country, so far from home.

Bronwyn had asked Trevor if he wanted her to contact my children and give them an update and he said he would really appreciate if she could. There was some crossing of wires though, because Bronwyn thought Kristy knew and that she was just going to give her the latest update. However, this was not the case at all, and poor Bronwyn was put in an awkward position due to this very understandable misunderstanding.

Because Trevor's children and mine live apart from each other, they had never really gotten to know each other, so there were a lot of things about each other's lives that they didn't know. I have always been grateful for the love and respect Trevor's children, their partners and the grandchildren have shown me and he feels the same about mine. We both accept each other's children and offspring and love them as though they were our own.

My son, Steven was living with Kristy in Townsville, North Queensland, so Bronwyn only needed to make one call. Despite having offered to do it, as you can imagine, she wasn't looking forward to making the call. She had no idea of what their reaction would be to her and she didn't know what supports might be there for them if they needed any.

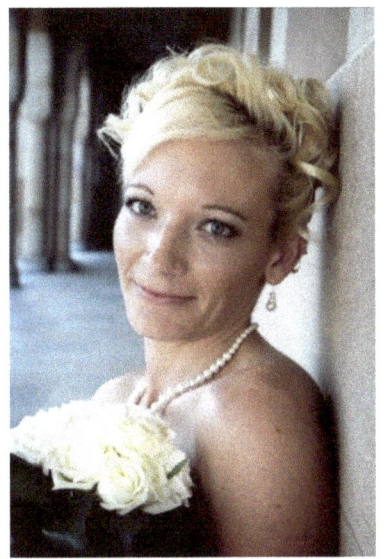

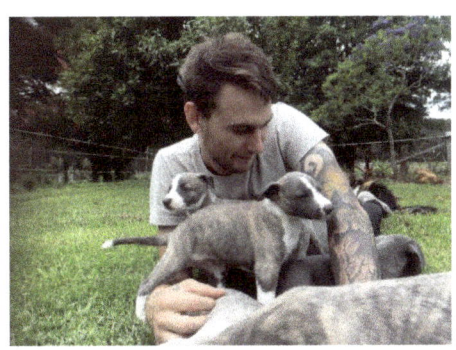

Kristy and Steven.

To put this call into context, the day before, Kristy had received a call from a telemarketer at 5am. As you might imagine, this did not bode well for the telemarketer, who was given short shrift.

The next day, the day Bronwyn was ringing, Kristy had set her alarm for 6.30am and, loving her sleep, wasn't too impressed when the phone raucously interrupted the last vestiges of peaceful slumber once again. Just like on the previous day, it was a call from overseas (she didn't know it was from Canada and could be Bronwyn trying to contact her), so she simply hung up.

Next thing she knew there was a text message on her phone from Bronwyn saying she'd just tried to call and wanted to give her an update on me and was there another number she could reach her on.

Well, this sure woke her with a real start and, so as not to disturb her partner, Kristy quietly went out of the bedroom and phoned Bronwyn straight back.

'Hi Bronwyn! It's Kristy here, Maya's daughter. What news? I haven't heard any news, let alone an update. What are you talking about?'

Her head was in a whizz!

She checked the clock and saw it was only 5.30am.

'Oh my God,' she thought. 'What's happened to Mum?'

'What was this 'news' Bronwyn was talking about? I haven't heard anything. She's on a cruise in Africa. Why, what's happened?'

Kristy's first thought, other than why was Bronwyn the first to hear news about me rather than her, was that I had contracted coronavirus. She'd been watching the news, and this was starting to get a bit more focus, so it was a natural assumption for her to make.

Because the internet is very sporadic on the ships, I have always told my children not to expect to hear from me until my return. I also hadn't written to them because, up until that point, we didn't have any answers and I didn't want to worry them needlessly. Also, I figured that when I got home, I would be able to phone them and tell them myself.

Although I didn't want to worry them then or now, I knew that they needed to be told because things were getting bad, and they were getting bad quickly. At this rate I knew that I might never see them, touch them or hold them in my arms again. It was hard, knowing that they were going to be receiving this news about me. I knew without a doubt that they would be devastated and really worried. I also knew that after hearing the news, that they would be thinking about, and trying to put in place a plan of how they could best support me in the gruesome journey that lay ahead for me.

I sent lots of love across the miles to them in the only way I could – silently and from my heart.

Bronwyn said: 'I'm so sorry, Kristy but they've only just found out that your mum has a brain tumour. They don't know much more than that and will let you know more as soon as they can. Your mother has lost her ability to talk properly so it's really hard for her to communicate. Tony [Bronwyn's husband] and I will do everything we can to support them and if you need anything, you can contact me anytime.'

Bronwyn then gave Kristy all the details of the hospital I had been admitted to, as well as her own details. She also gave her Trevor's phone number (the one he was using in Richards Bay), so she could also phone him direct.

Mark, her partner saw her distress and asked what was wrong to make her this upset. He listened to her as she told him as much as she knew at that time. Thank God he was there to give her some comfort and they both decided they would not tell Steven or her children until later that evening.

Next thing, her twin boys, Jake and Liam came into her room really excited. They were having their swimming carnival later that day and told her the school was using the swimming carnival to raise money for good causes.

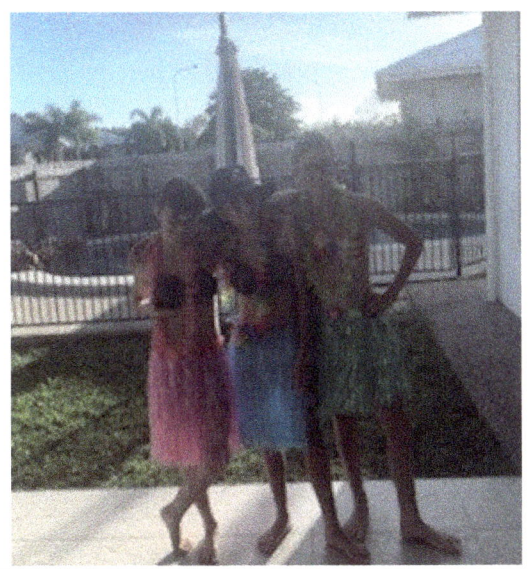

My grandsons off to the swimming carnival.

There were four house teams, and each house had its own special cause. They were very proud to tell her that this year, they were going to help raise money for brain cancer. They wanted some money to donate because the teachers had given all the children information about the importance of research and the way money was used to help save lives and increase the quality of lives for people with various disabilities and diseases, in this case, brain cancer. The boys had been really touched by the talks at school and were going to donate some of their own pocket money as well.

If she could have, and if it would have made a difference for me, Kristy would have given them everything she owned.

However, at this stage, she hadn't even broached the subject with her boys that I was diagnosed with a brain tumour. She had only just heard it herself and was still trying hard to process it all.

She gave the boys some money and got the three younger ones organised for school.

After this, she got ready and went to work.

She immediately rang the hospital and, being the middle of the night over there, she had lots of difficulty with the connection and answers that were not forthcoming. Eventually she did get onto them and the hospital was really concerned about getting a letter of guarantee from my private health and travel insurance so they could formally admit me.

Nothing was going to happen until all the paperwork was done.

Kristy, knowing her expertise in organising things, realised this was an area she could really help us with. She phoned Trevor and got the go-ahead as well as all the information she would need to help us with the travel insurance. She asked about my GP and our insurance company and then got to work phoning everyone to get things moving.

It was quite a difficult task to co-ordinate all of this, with her being in Townsville, my doctor in Bulahdelah, the insurance company in Sydney, Trevor in a lodge in Richards Bay and me in the emergency ward. It wasn't just a matter of co-ordination and approval, we had to have this letter of guarantee faxed or emailed to the hospital prior to them doing anything else for me.

While she was co-ordinating all of this (taking up several hours out of her very busy day), she also consulted Google about my diagnosis, prognosis, and likely outcomes and was also researching and checking up on Dr. Timakia. She wasn't going to allow just **anyone** to look after me. She was concerned about me being in South Africa, getting medical treatment there and she wanted to be sure he was good enough at his job and had the skills to look after me in the way she would like. She was scared I would die in this place, a place that in her mind was way behind the times.

Little did she know what fabulous hands I would be in – such blessed, healing hands.

When she did get through to the hospital, she asked if she could speak to me. A nurse came to me and told me my daughter was on the phone. She asked me to come to the reception area because she did not want to lose the connection and couldn't transfer the phone. I was so excited that I would be talking to her, but I was also really nervous because of my inability to talk.

I didn't know what she would be expecting, and I was scared it would be a one-way conversation and I wouldn't be able to communicate. Also, Trevor wasn't there as my go-between. I knew I wouldn't be able to explain things to her verbally as I would have done in the past. I realised, too, how different it is when you speak to someone over the phone. You have no body language to look at and when the other person has problems with their wording, e.g. finding words, huge pauses and blanks in conversations, these are only magnified. Also, the intonation can so easily be misconstrued and what might be just a matter of getting thoughts together for one person can sound from the other end like a lack of understanding. I should have had more faith in my girl.

I knew she was not able to see the joy on my face at hearing her voice. She just heard the tears in my voice and misunderstood these as tears of sadness. I just wanted her sitting beside me so I could hold her hand and we could just be. I knew that if this had been the case, she would have seen that I wasn't upset for me and that I truly wasn't scared. By the end of the conversation, I think she did know this.

She started by saying: 'Mum, Bronwyn rang and told me what's going on. I am so sorry, Mum. I know you can't talk, so I'll do most of the talking. I've called Trevor and he gave me the travel insurance details. I am happy to sort all of that out for you, so you don't have to worry about that. I wish I was there with you. I love you so much and if there's anything else you want or need, let me know.'

What a relief it was that she was the one to talk first and seemed to have grasped the situation so succinctly. I said a silent prayer for Bronwyn for finding the right words when telling her and I also thanked God once again for Trevor who also reiterated what Bronwyn had told her (several hours later but prior to her phoning me – time changes, remember).

I couldn't find words. Here was my 39-year-old baby girl, the light of my life, really upset because of what was happening to me. I wanted to spare her from this grief but knew I couldn't. I wanted her life to just go on as before without the worry about me, but I couldn't. I wanted to spare her any extra work, like sorting out the insurance company, but I couldn't, partially because I really couldn't, but also because I thought that putting this extra stress on Trevor would just tip the scales. He hates paperwork at the best of times. Besides, even if he wasn't the one who was wading through the whole maze of paperwork that was likely to ensue, he would have still have to do his share of liaising with them in any case.

So, Kristy had very kindly offered and given her fantastic organisation and business skills, I was glad to give consent to the insurance company when they rang.

Trevor had already paid $AU12,000 up front for my on-board hospital bill and my medical tests up to this point and he knew this was only the beginning … and I hadn't even moved out of the emergency department.

He seemed to be continuously handing over his credit card for one procedure after another, one test after another and he could visualise his credit card being stretched so far it resembled over-blown bubble gum – he knew there was not much stretch left in it, and he might end up with it splattered all over his face.

He knew our budget was not going to stretch much further and after coming to the harsh reality that there was nothing he could do, he decided to just pay and pay and pay until someone actually told him he'd reached his limit and then leave it in the lap of the gods. What else could he do?

He had no plan B. Interestingly though, when you know there is nothing else you can do, you often discover exactly what faith is all about. He just had to pray and believe that our claim would be accepted.

It didn't help that the hospital was so difficult to deal with and didn't seem to understand what was required of them to make it all happen. They kept asking for the letter of guarantee so they were assured of full payment, but they didn't send the appropriate paperwork to ensure this could happen. It was like they were at cross-purposes with the insurance company, even though they were all supposedly on the same page.

Kristy and Trevor were ready to pull their hair out initially because the hospital just kept asking them the same questions, questions that both Kristy and Trevor had already answered. Every five minutes or so, they'd get a call because the insurance company weren't getting the right information so, in the end, the insurance company just took control and really took them (the hospital) to task to ensure I would be covered.

It was thanks to Trevor and Kristy's diligence, our GP, Dr. Naal Hussain's prompt response to them regarding my previous impeccable medical history and the insurance company's persistence, that everything was approved.

This meant that as soon as a bed was available, I would be transferred to the ICU, or did it?

Kristy told me later she went for a long run early that morning while the kids were getting ready for school and their swimming carnival. She needed a bit of alone time so she could process the news that had just come out of the blue. She didn't know what to do. Part of her was angry that this could happen to me, and she just wanted to lash out at this unfair God who let these things happen.

That evening, she told Steven and her children. She didn't go into too much detail and she let them ask her any questions as time went on. She has always been very honest with her children, but she was also very aware that she didn't want them worrying to the degree that she was.

Kristy and Steven had worked together that day and she said it was really hard to avoid him as she made countless calls trying to put things in place for me. However, she just couldn't cope with having to be the bearer of this news to her brother, 10 years her junior, without first getting all of the facts for herself and knowing everything that could be in place, was.

She felt this deep, inexplicable rage well up inside with her feelings bubbling up at the most inopportune times like a volcano just waiting to erupt. She had no option but to bottle all of this in though, because, like me, she tends to be seen as the strength in her family and she believed if she gave into these feelings, it would make it so much more difficult for her children to cope.

She knew it was a matter of working through it on her own first and then to try to tell her boys in a calm, rational manner.

She found it such a blessing that her work, as director of Sparkles Cleaning Agency in Townsville, gave her the physical outlet she so much needed. At every opportunity, she would redirect all of this inexplicable rage she felt into her work and in dealing with sorting out and getting things moving at the hospital.

Despite all she was contending with, she never lost her cool with anyone, (especially the hospital), but I know her level of frustration at this stage was pretty high. If she'd lost her cool, she knew it might adversely impact our situation. She had to hold all of this inside.

Steven, when she told him, was very quiet, as is often his way, especially when things touch him deeply. Although both my children are very sensitive, Kristy has a real fire in her belly and tackles everything head-on. Steven, on the other hand, is a little more reserved, needs more time to process things and has difficulties showing his real feelings and this time was no exception. I didn't want to put any pressure on him. I had no doubts that my children and Trevor's children were all there for us and would move Heaven and Earth to help us, as they did.

Trevor arrived at the hospital about 9am, expecting to see me in ICU and was surprised to see me, in my pink dress that I'd had on the day before, still in the emergency department. At this stage I'd already been in there for almost 24 hours.

I had tried to get a nurse's attention during the night to find out what was happening and when they were going to transfer me, but every time I tried, they were either really busy, or I could not make myself understood.

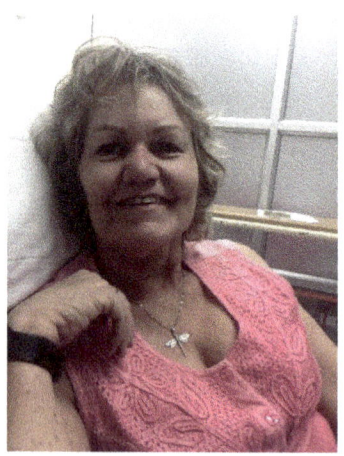

Me, waiting in the emergency department

The other complication was, that although everyone can speak English, their first language is Xhosa (pronounced Kossa), Afrikaans and Zulu. Xhosa was the most amazing language – one I certainly couldn't get my tongue around (even if I could speak properly). The tongue makes a clicking sound in the back of the throat, like a staccato beat, while the mouth forms the actual words. This was the most popular language I heard, and it was totally unintelligible to me. All their handovers were done in this mother tongue as well.

When Trevor walked in that morning and saw the way I was looking at him with a serene, almost peacefully detached look on my face, the light and sparkle gone from my eyes, the decline in me again hit him full-on. He realised at this point everything was now squarely on his shoulders.

He said it was like I was in the eye of the storm.

There was chaos and drama all around me. There was money for tests to be paid up front, more tests to be done and paid for, people to be contacted, phone credits to be sorted, doctors to see, travel insurance to be sorted, people to be organised to look after the farm, me to be transferred to intensive care, taxis to be organised for transfer to and from the hospital and the port agent to be contacted and liaised with. All the while, there I was sitting in my little safe cocoon, seemingly oblivious to everything going on around me that was threatening every aspect of our lives and ready to take me away and leave Trevor cleaning up the destruction in its aftermath.

I did know the facts of what he was dealing with, but for me it was like reading a horror story that you're not really a part of. I was the main character, but it was like I could pick up or leave the book at any time and I was not scared by the story line.

It was a surreal situation, but on some level, my detachment made it easier on Trevor, because the last thing he needed at this time was a repeat performance of my behaviour and reaction of the day before when I'd been consumed with fear and anxiety.

This state of mind continued, and although it was partly due to the drugs the doctor had commenced me on (Dexamethasone – to reduce swelling and Epilim – to reduce the risk of seizures), it was mainly because of where the tumour was located and the fact that this part of my brain was becoming even more impacted by the minute.

Even when not suffering a brain tumour and in my normal state, people know me as a very positive, inspiring person and this was something that helped me through some of the tough days, weeks and months that were ahead of me.

It's difficult to explain the intensity that Trevor felt and the juxtaposition of all that was on his mind and the emptiness in mine. That time while we were waiting in the emergency room was so intense because everything was happening at once and nothing was happening, all at the same time. Every time we asked about when I was going to be moved, the various staff we asked said: 'It won't be long now.'

That was said so many times we lost count and it wasn't until after I was moved up to intensive care that we understood what the delay was all about.

To get me into intensive care, a specific bed needed to become available. Due to my high risk of infection pre- and post-operatively (if they chose to operate), I needed a room that was glassed in with triple air filters in the air-conditioning ducts. They had to sterilise the room and move patients around, sterilising as they went.

Finally, after 30 hours in the emergency department, everything was ready and I was on my way. At 3pm, one of the nurses wheeled me on the narrow bed that was mine since admission to intensive care. We went into the lift and up to the fourth floor, turned right and went through the security doors to what was to be my new home for the next few weeks. I was moved onto a wider, much more comfortable bed, in a fully enclosed large glass room. There were only four beds like this in the entire two wards that comprised the ICU. All the others were just cubicles with curtain barriers between the beds.

I was allocated a nurse who hooked me up to some of the monitoring machines. Then she opened up this huge piece of paper (when unfolded created at least four A4-sized sheets). She spread this out, took more of a history, taking notes as she went. This was the way their paperwork looked. Being a nurse myself, I thought: 'How cumbersome and how difficult it must be to continually have to open it all up and then fold it all together.'

It seemed messy ... and what about all the crease lines?

Obviously, it worked well for them and having it set out this way meant everything was on full view every time they opened my file to check my progress. 'Maybe it's not such a bad idea after all,' I thought.

After Trevor had settled me in my new environment, he said he needed to go back to the Indaba Lodge. It was already 4pm and he'd spent most of the day with me.

On his return there, he knew there was much to do.

He needed to let Tristan know that Dr. Timakia was going to send all the information to him, and also to Bronwyn.

He needed to organise getting the person who was looking after our farm to extend his stay. Unfortunately, Warren couldn't do this due to other commitments, but Kristy again saved our bacon. She contacted a couple who had minded the farm several times before, Petra and Wolfgang, and they dropped everything and immediately came up to do whatever was needed. Even though they had other commitments, they quickly altered these and came to our aid. They were only able to stay until March 13, but we figured if we needed to stay in Richards Bay any longer, we would cross that bridge when we came to it. Petra and Wolfgang showed us the meaning of being there when it counts and for that we were and are eternally grateful.

Kristy also continued to work through the maze of bills and was in constant contact with the hospital and with Cover-More Travel Insurance, either by phone or email.

Once the initial paperwork and screening was complete, the hospital and Cover-More interactions were seamless. Not once did the insurance company question one bill or one decision made by the hospital. They also contacted us every day, asking how I was and showed genuine interest in me.

We knew we were in good hands and felt safe, secure and looked after, despite being so far from home and so far from everyone dear to us.

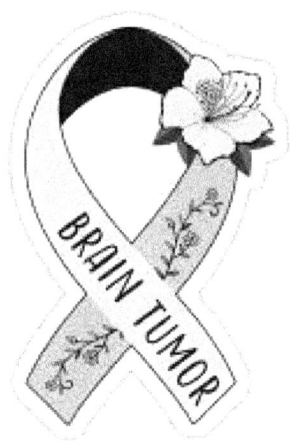

When you grow weaker,
Know that this is only in your body.

Your soul remains timeless
And this is what will carry you through
The debilitating factors before you.

Embrace each of these
As tests upon your spirit
And know with certainty
That you must not ever give up
On yourself,
Your true, authentic self.

CHAPTER 11

Wednesday, February 19

I got used to life in intensive care very quickly. I wasn't physically sick, and I had no pain. All my physical observations including my blood pressure, pulse and temperature remained stable throughout. It was hard to believe that I was actually as sick as I was, and that the threat of me dying remained a very real possibility. This was the truth of it and this thought was never really far from our minds.

We had discussed our views on death and life after death on quite a number of occasions and having a deep spiritual belief helped, so neither of us feared it. The thing we did fear was all that could happen before the final transition and this was still something we could not predict.

We had both heard many horror stories of people with brain tumours and with Fred showing himself so aggressively, as well as his relentless pursuit in taking control of my motor and communication skills, leaving me weaker and less co-ordinated by the day, made us wonder what else he had in store for me before he might take over completely.

I remembered reading a book several years ago about a woman who was dealing with early onset dementia called

Who Will I Be When I Die and I realised that all the questions and thoughts she had weren't too dissimilar to my own.

My mother had been diagnosed with dementia when she was in her late 80s and, in many ways, it had come as a bit of a blessing to her.

She had always feared living on her own and when Dad died (three years before her), although she knew on some level he had died, on another level she was happy in her own little world and didn't miss him as we all feared she might.

I would look at her in the last few years prior to her death and she just radiated love and peace. People were drawn to her and loved doing things for her because she showed so much gratitude. This was especially good to see when she'd deteriorated to the point where she needed to be transferred to a dementia ward.

Because of her peaceful and loving demeanour, we knew and felt confident that the nurses always gave her the best care. It's human nature really. When you have to look after someone who is cantankerous or aggressive, we all try to avoid it. But when someone makes us feel appreciated and isn't demanding, it becomes a pleasure to go the extra mile for them. She was also very patient with her co-patients and could often settle them down much easier than the staff could. Everybody loved her because of her kindness and gentleness and although she didn't recognise us from time to time, she always greeted us with the most welcoming smile.

In our years growing up, my parents were not very demonstrative in their feeling towards my brothers and sister and me, but in the years prior to mum's death, she made up for this. She always held my hand, hugged me and smothered me in kisses. She laughed a lot and often this was at herself.

I remember one time she had been transferred from the dementia ward to a hospital ward with a heart complaint. She was really sick, had a high temperature and had difficulty breathing. The medical staff had trouble getting her temperature down and we thought she was very close to death.

I had travelled up to Brisbane thinking this could be the last time I would see her. One day I was by her bedside and said to her: 'Mum, you don't need to hang on any longer. If you want to go, Dad is waiting on the other side for you.'
She said: 'Well, he can just wait a bit longer, because I'm not going anywhere.'
Well, that was sure telling me!

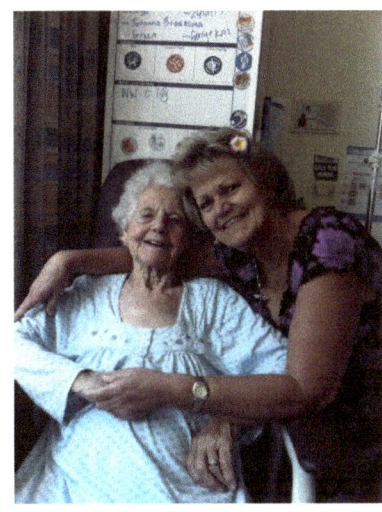

Visiting Mum, when she was very sick in hospital.

She lived another 18 months after that.

While I was in hospital in Richards Bay, my mother was never really far from my thoughts.

It was a funny sensation, but as the week went by, I started to feel her spirit resting within me and, when I looked at myself in the mirror, I could often see her image reflected back to me.

Trevor and my brother, Hans (who saw videos of me during this time) commented on this as well.

Part of it was the vacant look I had on my face a lot of the time as though I was in La-La Land, but another part, I believed, was her letting me know that she was with me and would always be there for me, giving me strength to fight whatever was ahead.

We had been very close in the adult years of my life and had always had a very definite, spiritual connection. While in hospital, even though she wasn't there, this connection seemed to become stronger, and it was of real comfort to me. It helped get me through some of the darker times – the times when my negative thoughts would encroach upon the positive outlook I had for the most part.

The final chapter in my book, *Emails From Heaven* came to my mind over and over as well and it reminded me of the way I wanted to be remembered, regardless of how many days, weeks, months or if I was lucky, years I had ahead of me.

From Emails From Heaven 2019
by Maya Knight

To be remembered is to leave an indelible impression
On someone whose heart, mind and very soul
Has been touched by you.

Material things are transient.
Money never lasts very long.
Promises not kept become defaults

And a life lived in selfishness
Is just a disaster in the end.

It is often the smallest things that leave
The biggest indentation ... The ripple effect.

It is our virtues that people remember.
And the virtues I speak of
Are Faith, Hope and Charity

To give someone a lifeline
When they are bereft and without an anchor.
To show someone a light
When darkness has overshadowed them.
To give of yourself, and to give freely
With no thought of recompense.
These, which add up to love,
Are what we are remembered for

To leave a legacy is just like leaving a footprint in the sand,
The tides and time wash them away.
But when you leave an indelible footprint on the heart,
Soul to soul, it lasts forever

I believe that if we are remembered for love

Then we are remembered for the greatest of all qualities,
Because it's love that oils the wheels of human joy.

I wanted to be remembered for love just like we remembered my mum, not as the woman who had dementia and often couldn't remember who we were, but as the beautiful woman she was, who lived, laughed and loved.

I realised the importance of love and I wanted to make my mum proud as I made this my mission for the life I had in front of me.

I found being loving such an easy thing to do. People around me were so amazing and so thoughtful and kind. Nothing was too much trouble.

As the number of days in the ICU started to increase, so did my decline mentally and physically.

Trevor came every morning about eight o'clock and usually stayed until three in the afternoon, when his driver (organised by Princess Cruises) would come and pick him up and take him home to Indaba Lodge, about a twenty-minute drive from the hospital.

Having a visitor in an intensive care ward for such long hours is usually not the done thing, but I think the staff realised the gravity of our situation, plus the fact that we were in this strange land with none of the usual supports around us.

As a culture, we observed a real closeness in families, not just immediate families, but extended families as well. There was a high regard and respect shown to older people and from what we observed, there was a spiritual belief that seemed to hold people together, not through fear, but through love, sharing, caring and support.

This was something that I really felt throughout my stay. Trevor often commented on this as well.

In the week prior to my operation, the strength in my upper right side became less and less, to the point where holding anything in my right hand became nigh on impossible.

I needed help with eating because, not only could I not hold a utensil in my right hand, the right side of my face was also affected and had a very definite droop. I looked like I'd had a mild stroke and the effects of the tumour were the same as if I'd suffered a mild stroke except for the fact that I still had normal strength in my lower limbs.

Having said that though, co-ordination of tasks was a little erratic. It took me a lot longer to do things because it became more difficult to think, prioritise and multitask.

It was a good thing that everything for my shower was laid out for me in the morning by the nurses and that it only comprised towels and a gown to wear. My toiletries were my own and were reduced to a small zip-up, waterproof case that included some soap, a washer, shower cap, my face cleanser and some moisturiser. I also had some basic foundation, blusher and lipstick, for special occasions (because everyday you're alive is a special occasion).

I did have some clothes in my locker, and although initially it was just what I'd walked into the hospital wearing, as well as a few undergarments, my wardrobe did increase a little, because Trevor bought me the most beautiful authentic Zulu skirt, necklace and earrings.

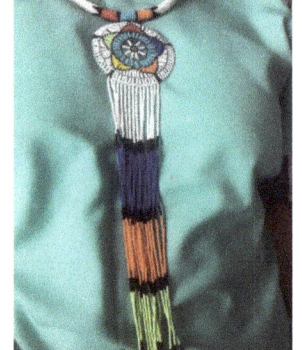

I was so lucky having the room that I did. There was a full wall of windows and I loved having the curtains left open so I could tell when a new day was about to burst forth. Although I missed seeing sunrises or sunsets because of the aspect of the room, I certainly knew when dark started to be filled with light heralding another new day. I had a great view of the shopping centre car park as well as the Kentucky Fried Chicken store, just across the road.

Although not being a lover of fast foods, the temptation of having a Kentucky Fried Chicken fast food store right there, beckoning me to indulge my taste buds in their culinary delights, was just too much.

The morning menu in the hospital, although often lukewarm, was quite appetising with oatmeal, bacon, eggs and toast and tea and juice. It was the highlight of the hospital cuisine.

However, things certainly went downhill from there with very little variety and everything covered in gravy (something I don't particularly like). The choices were chicken or meat plus potato or rice and one vegetable. The other alternative was fish (the better option as far as I was concerned).

So, seeing this across the road every day, I started to drool at the thought of french fries and a yummy zinger burger. Even though I had to be fed by Trevor, I enjoyed every morsel of it. And this time, I had a legitimate reason for being a little messy in my eating habits.

My days started to have a very definite routine that revolved around getting up, showering, eating, having my medications intravenously and orally, Trevor being with me most of the day, having regular rests and watching a bit of television.

I was unable to write, and reading was also impossible because I couldn't hold a book properly and I couldn't concentrate on anything for too long because it would hurt my brain.

I have always loved my showers and it's always where I've done my best thinking. I have had so many epiphanies in the shower in the past and I see this as my 'special place'.

The nurses, although giving me lots of independence, were also close at hand if I needed some assistance.

There was only one shower and toilet combined for the ward and it was on the other side of the ward, meaning I had to walk out of my room, past four cubicles and through another set of doors and then into the shower area. I usually had my shower early, way before anyone else, because that way I would not feel too pressured and feel I had to rush. There was a chair in the shower, and I would regulate the water and then sit as I lathered myself and rinsed off. It always felt so nice to start the day fresh and clean. There was an emergency buzzer but fortunately I didn't need to use it ever. Getting dressed wasn't too much of an ordeal but getting my shoes on and off proved a bit more difficult.

One thing I found particularly difficult was when I'd been lying in bed (usually during the night) and needed to go to the toilet, *quickly!*

Firstly, I had to extrapolate myself from everything I was wired up to that was monitoring my vital signs. Fortunately, the nurses were close by and were very adept at this. Then I would try to wriggle down to the bottom of the bed, co-ordinate my legs over the side, place my feet to the ground, position my shoes so my feet could slip into them easily and then slide into them without pushing them away.

Everything became really difficult because every task in the past that I had taken so much for granted, I now realised was broken down into so many different parts and at that time my brain had difficulty putting these in order and doing them automatically.

Trevor was absolutely amazing. He never once complained about my inability to do things and he was there for me in whatever capacity I needed. He would come in with the news of the day, telling me about people he'd contacted and their responses as well as what was happening in the world.

It was just so easy to have him there. I felt I could rest if I wanted to, and he would get us both a coffee, or just get one for himself if I didn't want one.

Sometimes the nurses needed to do something with me, so he would just make himself scarce at those times.

When I rested, he would often read. He found a good book shop in the shopping centre and was a regular customer there and at the café, the bank (to exchange money) and the phone shops to buy extra credit.

He went into one of these shops one day and happened to get chatting with the manager of the store, Sharmilla. Usually, she didn't work front of shop but for some reason, she was there. Being Caucasian, we were the minority in this country of many cultures and colours (the rainbow nation). Also, she hadn't seen him before, so being a good people person, she got into a conversation with him and asked him if he was on holidays. Trevor briefly told her about our situation and why we were in Richards Bay. He bought what he needed and was also assisted with a few other things and thought that would be the end of that.

That evening, a young woman stood at my doorway and asked me if my name was Maya and if I was married to Trevor Knight. I nodded, not knowing who she was or what she wanted. She told me that Trevor had been into the shop earlier and for the rest of the day she hadn't been able to get me out of her mind. She wanted to know if it was okay if she visited with me. Of course it was okay, so I nodded. Trevor hadn't mentioned it because he didn't think it had been significant – just someone in passing. How wrong he was.

She brought me the most beautiful vase with three roses and although not usually allowed in the intensive care area, I was indulged and was permitted to have it on my windowsill for the next twenty-four hours, after which time they put it in the nurses' station where I could admire it from afar.

She also brought me slices of fresh fruit. I just wanted to hug her to bits for that. It had seemed like ages since I'd had that taste of clean, fresh fruit. It was just so thoughtful and kind.

I can't explain what transpired between us. Here we were, total strangers from different parts of the world yet there was this strange affinity that neither of us could deny. She held my hands (despite her being a very private, not openly affectionate person) and we communicated more without words than verbally. It was like our hearts were connected and we both knew and felt it.

She became a regular visitor, coming early evenings when she'd finished work and would often spoil me with fresh fruit.

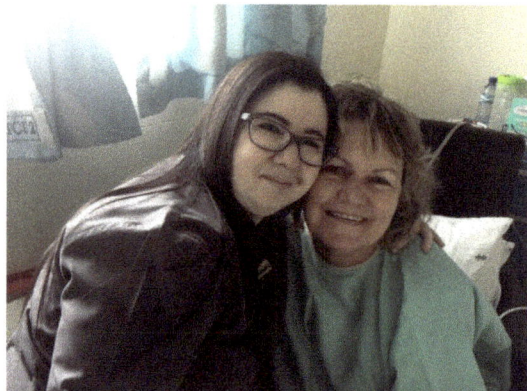

Shamilla and me before the operation.

We had other visitors as well and fortunately Trevor was with me when people came so he could keep people updated and speak for me when I couldn't.

I found it very difficult to respond the way I used to in any conversation because I could only hold onto the very last phrase of any conversation in my mind and respond to that. It was like that was all my brain could work with at the time. On another level I certainly retained full comprehension and understanding of everything that was said and what was going on around me.

I tried not to get frustrated, but at times it really did get the better of me. I started to sound like the old gentleman in *The Vicar of Dibley* saying: 'No! No! No! Yes! (but I would say sh*t!).' Obviously, I had developed a slight case of Tourette's syndrome by then as well …

I always knew how amazing Trevor was, but there were times when he amazed me even more. Nothing was too much trouble and, although I wasn't consciously demanding of him, I'm sure I did stretch his patience on many occasions. He was so devoted to me and was so committed to keeping everyone we knew and loved in the loop.

He constantly kept in touch with Bronwyn, Tristan and Kristy, thanking them for the incredible job they were all doing, each in their own way with their unique skill sets. He recognised, as did I, what an insurmountable task it would have been to get through this alone.

Remarkably, Dr. Timakia had been in constant contact with our children, including Kristy, keeping them abreast of my medical condition as well. However, he was in particularly close contact with Tristan (Trevor's pathologist son).

He emailed him, not only with all my medical information, but also all my MRI scans and results as well. Tristan examined these thoroughly using his trained medical and analytical brain.

Tristan phoned Trevor the day after I was admitted to the ICU and told him that from the scans, it looked like my tumour may not be as bad as was initially thought. He believed it was a meningioma – a tumour that arises from the meninges and not within the brain itself. The meninges are the membranous layers that cushion the central nervous system. The really good news though, was that 90 percent of meningiomas are benign.

Given the look of the tumour, its position close to the skull, and that I'd had no symptoms up until a few weeks prior, and that the symptoms were very much in keeping with those of a meningioma, it was a logical conclusion to make.

He discussed this with Dr. Timakia as well and, although it gave us a glimmer of hope, we wouldn't know for sure until either a biopsy was taken, or it was surgically removed, hopefully completely. Either way, there were still huge risks involved.

It constantly surprised us that Dr. Timakia was so willing to engage with Tristan and it showed us his real strengths as a person and as a doctor – someone we could totally depend on who would not put his ego ahead of our welfare.

Trevor made sure Tristan knew that he was held in very high esteem by the medical staff in Richards Bay and how reassuring it was to know that we didn't just have one single opinion to rely on anymore. He told him in his email that the phone call he'd had the day before was like a glimmer of light at the end of a very dark tunnel and that Tristan had pulled him out of a tailspin and put him back on course.

It had been a real shot in the arm and gave us hope.

When Trevor emailed Bronwyn, he reiterated what a rock she was to him in this very dark time. He was so grateful to her for initially informing people (our family and close friends) at a time when it had been too much for him to do and he made mention of the song he had written for her several years ago, little knowing how prophetic he was being at the time.

"We may worry about each other, but that's only 'cause we care,
You'll always have my shoulder every time.
We don't need to be together for me to know you're there,
You're a comfort in this crazy world of mine."

His emails always told each of our children how proud we both were of them and how dearly we both loved them and then he would get into telling them the practicalities of what was happening just to keep everyone updated.

He let them know that physically I remained well, and I was eating well (the only problem was actually getting the food into my mouth)!

He told them I was sleeping and moving around with no problems except for a lack of strength in my right upper side.

He told them that my thought processes were very confused, something the doctor had told him to expect, and that he had to play 'the guessing game charades' with me (for example: the day before, I had told him that it was too hot, and I needed him to turn the bed down. I was sitting in a chair at the time, so he obviously deduced I meant the air conditioner).

I have no recollection of this and there are probably many other things that I said to him that were strange that he had to try to decipher. However, my comprehension remained intact and this made our communication easier because I knew and understood everything he was saying to me.

Trevor let everyone know that even though Tristan's assessment of the situation was a very positive one, and although he and I had a really positive outlook, we had had a very frank talk about the alternative and I had reassured him that I was prepared for any outcome – even if it meant saying goodbye – I was ready.

Trevor told them how brave and courageous I was and how much he loved me and that this, as well as our love for each other is what fueled us both and that it would help both of us get through anything.

I had asked Trevor to take a photo of me every day because I wanted to have a record of my progress.

Thanks to the wonderful world of technology, we were also able to talk on WhatsApp and Facetime, so we could actually see those we loved so much as we talked to them. I think it also helped allay some fears for them as well, seeing that I actually looked quite well and had such a positive attitude.

Reception, at times, left a bit to be desired but overall, especially in my early days in intensive care, it was really good. Most mornings I got to talk to Bronwyn and Kristy (who would then update everyone else).

Trevor reassured each of them that both of us were now ready to face life head-on, only this time, he and I would be standing shoulder to shoulder with the three best people in our world, our main supports – Tristan, Bronwyn and Kristy.

He contacted the ship's agent from Grayboy in Australia, Elise to thank her for their phenomenal support and let her know the basic facts of the situation we were in. At this stage we knew for sure I had a huge tumour in my head, hopefully a benign meningioma and that I was in the best place with the best medical team possible. It was likely that my operation would be on Friday, February 21, but that depended on how quickly the swelling in my brain decreased.

We were both aware that life goes on and commitments need to be upheld and, as long as all went well, Trevor would be going on the next cruise as was scheduled (on his own, as obviously I was not well enough).

Kristy had been approved to fly over to Richards Bay to be with me and fly home with me when I was able. My insurance company was going to pay for the flights and amazingly, Princess Cruises offered to pay for her accommodation, meals and a driver whilst she was with me in Richards Bay.

Kristy sent an email back to Trevor and although it was very personal, I wanted to share most of it because it just reiterated to me the amazing woman she is.

She wanted us to know that they would all be there for us in any way we needed them to be – Kristy, Mark (her partner), Steven (my 28-year-old son) and my grandchildren, Jaydn (21), Matthew (13), and the twins, Liam and Jake (12).

She said she felt positive about the outcome but realised things don't always go the way you want, and she wanted to make sure we had this very real conversation.

She specifically asked Trevor to read out her email to me so we could then move forward honestly, realistically and positively as we have always done.

She wanted me to know the following:
- She would always have Steven's back because he is her brother, and she loves him very much and will do anything it takes to make sure he has the support he needs and that they **will** stick together.
- She said if the worst did come about and they were to lose me from their lives, they would remain close to Trevor – if that's something he wanted. She wanted me to know that he is, and always will be, a big part of

their family. Also, she wanted me to know that they would give him any support he needed (as family does).

- She said they would not allow losing me to tear them apart, rather they would make it bring them closer together as I would wish.
- In essence, she promised to live life as an individual and as part of a family in a way that would make me proud.

She said she had so much hope that I would get through this because, to her, I am an inspiration, and as Trevor said so often, such a strong, courageous woman, and if anyone could get through this, she knew I could.

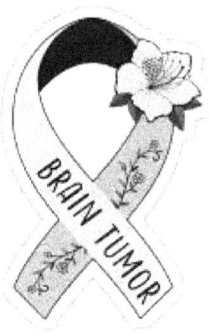

When you are most in need
Do not contemplate your misery.
Instead, place the emptiness
At the gates of opportunity.

Do not ask for the impossible
But expect that all will be provided.

Offer yourself completely
To what is required of you,
With no concern as to the outcome.

Trust fully and immerse yourself
In the here and now
And want for nothing
Except to be secure in your own cocoon
Of acceptance.

CHAPTER 12

Friday, February 21

I had been in the ICU for four days now and although things had settled down somewhat, we were far from being out of the woods. Perhaps we were just getting used to the routine and we knew that everything that needed to be done was being done.

The angst of being all by ourselves in a strange country had left us and was now replaced by this wonderful feeling of acceptance and belonging.

We still weren't sure whether Dr. Timakia was going to do an exploratory operation or whether he was going to bite the bullet and just take Fred out completely.

Trevor had had some very frank conversations with him and as far as Trevor was concerned, he needed to make it very clear he had the utmost faith in Dr. Timakia's ability and certainly realised the severity of my situation and would not hold him accountable should things go wrong.

Trevor had signed a DNR at their very first meeting and was very realistic as to the outcome of any surgical intervention.

We cannot begin to imagine the pressure Dr. Timakia must have felt. He actually wanted to do a biopsy and then get me on a plane home, thinking that this might be the best scenario.

However, from our point of view, this concerned us because we knew that the flight to Sri Lanka had probably exacerbated the tumour and started the bleed into my brain.

There were so many considerations and Dr. Timakia must have felt very torn. In some ways, us being from Australia would have complicated the decision- making process and I'm sure, that although he wanted what was best for me, the easiest option would be to send me home as soon as I was stable, and hopefully, sooner rather than later.

Not mincing any words, Trevor said quite bluntly: 'I'm not taking her home in a box and that's what will definitely happen if you don't operate. At least if you operate, it will give her the best chance she has.'

Trevor was very insistent, and I know only too well when Trevor sets his mind to something, there's no alternative and, what Trevor wanted was for me to be operated on in Richards Bay by Dr. Timakia– and that was that!

It was more than him just wanting things his own way, though. He knew in his gut that operating and taking Fred out in Richards Bay would be the only logical option and the only one that would give me the best chance of recovery, let alone life. He believed that to do anything less would be like putting a Band-Aid on a knife wound.

We know that Dr. Timakia really struggled with what was best for me. He had never personally come across a situation like ours before.

There were lots of issues he had to deal with; lots of hoops he had to jump through; lots of people who had a vested interest; lots of protocols he needed to adhere to.

And then there were all the personal demons that would have haunted him, making him wonder if he could do this successfully. Self-doubt would have been a constant companion in the days prior to my operation.

What if he failed?
What would be the repercussions to the hospital if it wasn't successful?
What were the repercussions to him personally as a doctor, especially treating a woman from another country?

Would he be held liable by my personal travel insurance if things didn't go according to plan?

And the list would have gone on and on and on.

There must have been so many things keeping him up at night, preparing him for what was expected of him.

Dr. Timakia consulted with his mentor on several occasions and together they went through the logistics of my operation and made sound preparations and strategies, taking everything into account including any problems that might be encountered.

He also contacted a very trusted colleague from Durban and asked him to be his wingman for the procedure.

He made sure Dr. Lucelle Padayochee was free as the anaesthetist and that the pathology department was ready to receive and examine the biopsy he would send them to determine exactly what it was he was removing. He wanted nothing but the best for me and he got the very best team of doctors and nurses together, not wanting to leave anything to chance.

Dr. Timakia had a discussion in layman's terms with Trevor and told him exactly what he was planning to do in the operation. He also let Kristy, Bronwyn and Tristan know (naturally giving it to Tristan in medical speak).

He then asked Trevor if they should do the operation with me awake or under anaesthetic.

Because various things they were planning to do might be very psychologically traumatic for me, Trevor said it would be best if I was out to it while they operated. He thought I would find it really difficult to cope with some of the things they would have to do, and on top of everything, experiencing them at the time could be very traumatic and could very much lead to PTSD (post-traumatic stress disorder) in the future. Not only would they have to drill holes into my skull, they'd need to do a full craniotomy where they would have to take out a huge part of my skull. As they did this, there would be a large flap of skin (my scalp) that they would have to put over my face out of the way.

In some ways, being under full anaesthetic can make brain surgery a little more difficult, because when the patient remains awake, the surgeon can stimulate certain areas of the brain and know which areas to avoid, and which are safe areas.

The brain is such an important and complex organ – in fact it's the most important organ in our entire body because it affects all we are and all we do.

Any injury, even minor, depending on where it occurs, can change our personality, our behaviour, as well as our ability to function.

The brain is made up of two hemispheres and each of these is made up of four lobes – frontal lobe, parietal lobe, occipital lobe and temporal lobe.

My tumour was in the left hemisphere of my brain in the left frontal and left temporal lobe region and, because it was so large (the size of a tennis ball), it was pushing the right hemisphere of my brain right over and squashing it. There was also considerable bleeding into my brain, and this complicated things even further.

The frontal lobe governs a number of things and the areas that were specifically affecting my brain were my level of consciousness, which showed up as vagueness. At times it was like the world was passing me by as I lay in this type of La-La Land.

It also affected my thinking and decision-making skills as well as my memory for things that had been habitual in the past, for example, the way I forgot how to use my phone.

I also had difficulty getting the order of things right, for example, unhooking all the tubes and monitoring equipment in the ICU when I needed to get up and either sit in my chair or go to the bathroom.

It became increasingly more difficult to focus, multitask and switch from one task to another. Processing information started to become an issue as well. I found that if there were multiple conversations at one time or there was a lot of information to process, I could only focus on a very small portion of it or on the last thing that was being said, especially if a response from me was required.

I was unable to bring into the front of my mind and respond with words, anything that wasn't immediate, even though I knew the gist of everything that had been said.

I could only cope with information given to me in small bite-sized pieces rather than in huge chunks.

Looking at me, people could certainly mistake my vague demeanour and communication difficulties for Alzheimer's, and although I did have difficulty accessing information at times, for example, when Trevor and Rowena were trying to look for our insurance details. The difference is that people with Alzheimer's have difficulty recalling and accessing recent memories, whereas I had full access to these, but it was like they were all jumbled up in a huge filing cabinet with no system for easy access and no logical or efficient means of individual retrieval.

The worst thing for me though, was my inability to express myself verbally. This was and always had been such a big part of 'me' and every day it seemed like more of 'me' was going. I couldn't find the right words to say, but if someone spoke them, I would understand exactly what they meant, as well as the emotion behind it.

This reminded me of my conversations with Mum and Dad. Although I was born in Holland, I have great difficulty speaking the language now. If needs be, I can do it though. However, it takes a lot of effort and doesn't come automatically. I have to say what I want to say in English in my head first, and then translate it to Dutch in my head before I say it out loud. It often meets with a lot of laughter because my pronunciation and grammar aren't the best. So, while my parents always spoke to me in Dutch (when there weren't any

English-speaking people around), I understood every single word and replied in English, something that worked for us and never seemed strange to us.

Even though my tumour was also in my left temporal lobe, the only real effects in this area seemed to be with my visual perception.

I found it very difficult to see people who weren't standing right in front of me. Although I was mostly very agreeable, and rarely got angry, I would get quite upset when people would stand or sit in my peripheral vision or to the side of me.

I knew full well that I could turn my head, but it seemed to hurt my brain to do so. I felt like it wasn't too much to ask, and it would certainly make a big difference to me, but all too often my request would be ignored because it did not seem significant.

Every time it happened, I got more and more irritated, and I started to think that people were doing it on purpose, although I know now that this certainly wasn't the case.

I remember one time when Dr. Timakia came to see me, and he stood just to the left at the end of my bed. I asked him to move to the middle at the end so I could see him properly, which he did, and then he moved again, ever so slightly, which really did annoy me. Let me just say that he certainly got the hint that I was a bit miffed (poor man)!

It's hard to explain exactly what it felt like for me. The only way I can explain it now is that it was like looking at someone who's standing totally out of your line of vision and although you know they're there, you just can't see them properly. Also, it was like looking through spectacles that are too strong for you, and instead of them helping you to focus, all they do is leave you with a headache and feeling sick in your stomach, especially if you move.

With everything I was experiencing, as well as Trevor's insistence and Cover-More Travel Insurance's blessings, it was accepted that the full operation was going to go ahead. Obviously, there really wasn't any choice.

This meant Dr. Timakia would have to do a craniotomy to open my skull and remove the tumour. A sample of the cells would then need to be sent to pathology to confirm the tumour type, as well as the grade of tumour.

Obviously, they were hoping, as were we, that the tumour would be benign, and they would be able to totally remove it. However, this would be unclear until the operation was well underway, and even if all went well and it was all removed and benign, there would still need to be extensive follow-up to ensure it did not re-grow. I would also need to be on medications to avoid my risk of seizures in the future. A lot would depend on the exact location of my tumour plus whether or not it was attached to any arteries or nerves.

Because I would be under full anaesthetic, Dr. Timakia and his team decided they would use a method called brain mapping. They used my MRI scans, which created a series of images of my brain in action and these images also captured the blood oxygen levels in the parts of my brain responsible for movement, perception, language and thinking. By identifying and mapping these eloquent areas, it then made it possible to remove my tumour to the greatest extent possible, without harming other areas. No wonder my MRI had taken so long and no wonder I had to go in for a second time. My thoughts were that they wanted to have everything ready if Dr. Timakia planned to do the operation using this brain-mapping technique. It was obviously the safest way to do my surgery and would be the least harmful to me and to my quality of life.

We had no idea at the time about everything that was going on prior to my operation, nor all of these preliminary preparations.

I think sometimes as a patient, it's all just taken for granted. However, this was a major operation with major risks and major implications should things go wrong.

While all of this was being prepared, Dr. Timakia also had his usual in-patient and outpatient clinics. He had other operations to perform, not to mention, a personal life to live with his beautiful, then eight-month-pregnant wife, Maya (what were the chances to have a wife with my name).

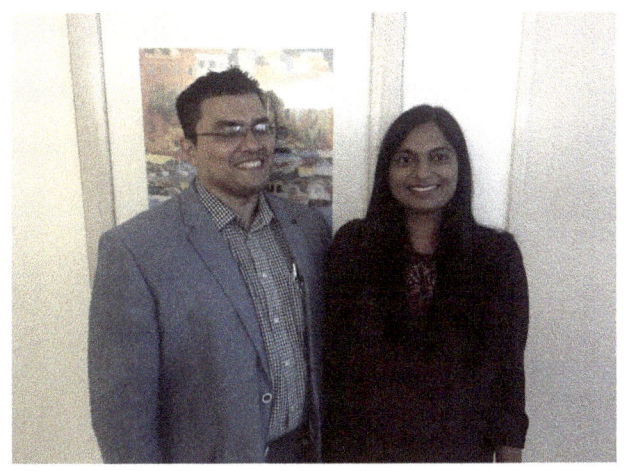

Dr. Timakia and his beautiful wife, Maya.

My operation was a bit of a change from the usual routine for him. The norm for him included spinal injuries and conditions, head injuries due to car accidents and gunshot wounds.

For Trevor, the list of people to contact started to increase as we realised how many lives intertwined with ours.

This was a really interesting exercise because if you'd asked me prior to this happening, I would have thought that our circle of family and friends who had a vested interest in our wellbeing and who cared about us was nowhere near as big as it became.

This of course meant the number of emails Trevor wrote or sent to multiple people increased and our phone credits were constantly in need of being topped up.

We had so many people who put us in their prayers and, strange as it may seem, we could feel the positive energy of their prayers. To say we felt blessed throughout our stay, is quite the understatement.

There were things that started to happen which were totally inexplicable and we started counting our blessings, rather than our misfortunes.

Trevor and I realised that our bond was becoming even stronger, and we were always conscious of each other's needs. I understood not to put too much pressure on him and to support him to get enough rest and, although I wanted him to see more of, and enjoy and venture into this gateway to so many safari parks, he wouldn't hear of it. He said the only place he wanted to be, was with me.

In one of the emails he sent to our dear friends, Ken and Margaret, he said: 'You can always see the true worth of a person when the chips are down and I am humbled by the strength and courage Maya is showing.'

He had faith that we would both get through this and be all the stronger for doing so.

The thing that really touched me, though, was that he said, 'I always knew I was married to an angel ... but in reality, she's a SUPER angel.'

His email to Phil Kaler, the head of entertainment at Princess Cruises, was a difficult one to write.

What do you say to someone representing such a big company who pulls out all the stops to help and support you? Words couldn't do justice to the gratitude we felt.

Just imagine if it were you, offloaded in a strange town in a strange land not knowing a single soul, not understanding some of the languages and having no means of transport, no accommodation, no adequate communication devices and then, on top of all this, hearing the sort of news we did.

The only way we really got through this from the very start to the day we got home was through the constant support from Princess Cruises.

We had our own port agent, Tamsin, who liaised by phone and in person, making regular visits to ensure all our needs were being met – mine and Trevor's.

This included finding and paying for his first-class accommodation, his meals, a driver to and from the hospital daily, plus so many incidentals including phone credits, not covered by our travel insurance.

These were things that were not required of them to do. After all, we were just contracted to work for the few weeks on board and if anything, we had broken our contract with them by needing to leave earlier. They owed us nothing.

Often people heading up big companies are seen as callous and heartless, but this was so far from our experience.

Although we have always been supported in so many ways by all the wonderful staff at Princess Cruises from the heads of departments through to the captain and every single one of the crew of every ship we have had the pleasure of sailing on, this went above and beyond anything we could ever have imagined and our gratitude knows no bounds.

When I was still in intensive care, the most beautiful bunch of flowers arrived at the Indaba Lodge for me along with lots of goodies. Unfortunately, the flowers weren't allowed in the ward, but Trevor took a photo to show me and brought in our little indulgence hamper, which we shared over the next few days. This really lifted my spirits and touched my soul very deeply.

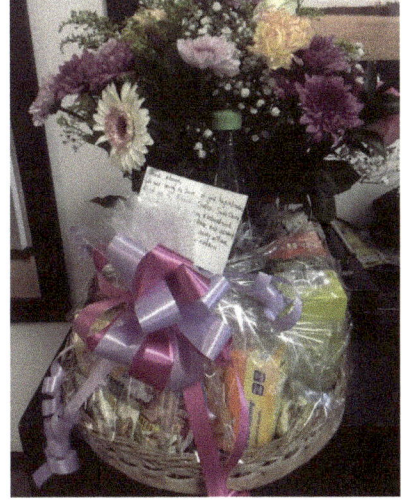

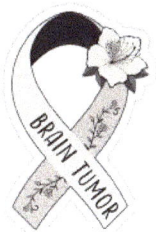

Life asked death,
"Why do people love me but hate you?"

Death responded,
"Because you are a beautiful lie and I am a painful truth."

— *Unknown*

CHAPTER 13

Monday, February 24

Today started like any other day with the sun rising about 5.30am. For so many people, this would just be another day, but it held great significance for me because this could well be my very last day ... ever.

However, despite the significance of it, it started just like most for me as well.

I'd had my shower, combed my blonde, shoulder-length hair (for the last time) and was patiently lying in my hospital bed all wired up, waiting for Trevor to arrive.

I was under no illusion as to what was in store for me today.

Trevor arrived about 7.30am and I was really happy to see him. We had grown extremely close over the last few days and we both had achieved such an easy way to be together.

We had looked death right in the eye; we had prepared for the fact that today might well be the beginning of the end, if not **the end;** we had made our peace and I had said everything I needed to say to Trevor and to those closest to me.

I didn't feel this urgency to talk as I might have thought I would. Trevor knew what was in my heart and I knew without a doubt what was in his, so waiting for my transfer to the operating theatre was not a time filled with angst.

Trevor took a video of us and, looking back on it, it was a very positive, though sad video. There was certainly no denying how deteriorated my condition had become. However, more than this, there was no denying the depth of love between us.

For some reason we did feel positive and believed that whatever was meant to be, would be, and it was all up to a power higher than us. There was no point in worrying, because as we had said so often in the previous days: 'Worry is just a down payment on fear,' and we certainly didn't want to go there. Also: 'What you focus on becomes your reality.'

The clock struck 12 (high noon) and it was time to be transferred to the pre-op room. To our great surprise, Trevor was allowed to go down there with me, walking alongside my hospital bed, wheeled by two wards-men. On arrival, a nurse from the ICU handed over all my relevant medical notes and gave a brief verbal handover to Dr. Lucelle Padayochee, my anaesthetist.

It was the first time I'd met her. She immediately captivated me with her intelligent, kind eyes and her soft and gentle demeanour. She instilled confidence in me even though I can't remember exactly what she said. I think she basically went through what was going to happen once I was in the operating theatre.

Sometimes it's not the words themselves that put people at ease, but the way they're said. Even Trevor doesn't recall what was said either; we both knew there was no hurry at this time, and that she was there for us and she would answer any last-minute questions we might have had at this time, honestly, and to the best of her ability.

I felt so safe in her care and knew without a doubt that having her and Dr. Timakia and the team they'd handpicked looking after me was the greatest gift I would ever receive.

When it was time for me to go through the theatre doors, Trevor said something to me that might seem very strange to all of you reading this. He said: 'Don't forget to look back because I'm going to be here, right up until you get on that plane. So, look back, Maya, because I'll be waving you goodbye!'

This really touched me so deeply, probably more than anything else he could have said. He made me smile and that's the way I left him, with love and joy in my heart and soul. In some way it helped me more than anything else did – this very special goodbye.

You see, it had always been a bit of a bone of contention for me that whenever Trevor was catching a flight to join a cruise ship and I wasn't going with him as he always seemed to be in such a rush to get through the departure gates at the airport. He wouldn't ever look back, despite the fact that I would always be standing by the window of the airport to say that final farewell as he was lost from my view.

Once I was in the operating theatre, I was briefly introduced to the team who were all gowned up and busy with their preparations. I was transferred onto the operating table and this was positioned allowing Dr. Timakia easy access to my head. I knew they would be clamping my head to keep it really rigid throughout the operation because the slightest movement could result in irreparable, permanent brain damage.

The first thing I noticed to my right as I lay there in wait, was my MRI scan showing my tumour – the size as well as the position. This was the very first time I'd actually seen it and I thought to myself: 'Oh my God ... it's huge! How on earth are they going to get all of that out? It's going to leave a huge cavity in my head!'

No sooner had I caught a glimpse of it, and one of the nurses quickly turned off the backlight behind it so I couldn't see it any longer ... but it was too late. Obviously, they didn't want me to see it and I can certainly understand why.

One might think that I would have felt very frightened and alone at this stage. There I was in this strange environment with all this strange equipment around me, Dr. Lucelle (as she'd asked us to call her) to my left, the operating team busy all around and Dr. Timakia nowhere in sight, but I was overwhelmed by this beautiful feeling of inner peace.

I didn't pray as such, but my heart was filled with overwhelming love and gratitude for all I'd had, all those I'd loved and those who'd loved me, all I'd experienced and for all I'd lived, and I knew there was no bigger prayer than that.

I looked in the eyes of those around me in that moment doing their best to save me and I said a silent 'thank you' as I drifted off ...

'Miracle in Richards Bay - Escape from the Vortex' by Maya Knight

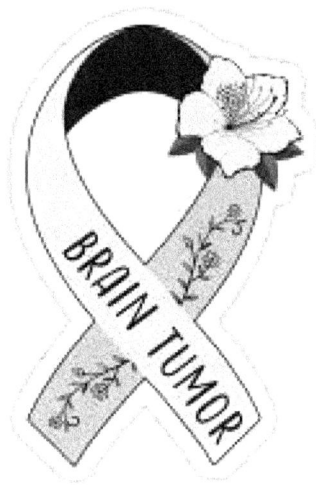

You must pray and believe
That all will come to you as you need it.

When steps are placed in your way
Know that they have been placed there
In order that you may learn
To climb to new heights

Your pain, though very real,
Is your test to once and for all
Create your own peace and tranquility.

CHAPTER 14

Then came the worst time of all – the waiting game.

Trevor went back to the Indaba Lodge and although the first few hours weren't too bad, this was only because he knew it would be a long operation (about eight hours, they thought). He had no expectation of hearing from the hospital within that time, so although his thoughts were never very far from me, he accepted that all was now in the lap of the gods.

The hospital staff had assured him they would call him if anything unforeseen happened and therefore, no news would be good news. Nonetheless, he wanted an update after a few hours – just to make sure things were all going according to plan. After all, they may have been trying to contact him and he may have been out of signal range. He felt a growing turmoil within him that he tried to quell. On the one hand he was really eager to hear news of how things were progressing, but on the other hand he didn't want to pester the staff there – after all they had enough to do. So, he practiced the virtue of patience.

By 8pm he was starting to get a bit antsy.

How was everything going? Were they finished yet? Did everything go well? Was it benign?

Questions! Questions! Questions!

Eventually he phoned the hospital. After all, the eight hours were nearly up. Unfortunately, at that stage there were no answers because they were still operating, so this meant more waiting.

Minutes after he rang, the operation was complete. Apparently, after hours of meticulously trying to remove my tumour without damaging any adjacent brain tissue, at the last moment, and to the surprise of the operating team, the remainder of my tumour just came away clean.

However, there was still a lot to do for and to me, and phoning Trevor was not the first thing on the hospital staff's agenda. They called him at 9pm to say I was back in ICU and that all went well. Although this was only an hour or so later, this final hour seemed the longest. As he sat and watched the second hand circumnavigating the clock face, he grew a little more anxious and the hints that all might not be as straightforward as he'd hoped were starting to gnaw at him.

When the phone rang and he saw it was the hospital, he held his breath until he heard those magic words: 'The operation has been successful.'

That was when he could finally let go of all the tension that had been building up in him, especially in that final hour. It seemed to explode out of him in a long breath of relief followed by quiet tears of gratitude for the skill of Dr. Timakia and Dr. Lucelle and the amazing operating team.

What a relief!

Finally, he could relax, knowing I had gotten through it, I was alive and I was being well looked after.

He knew that this meant I was now in an induced coma. We had both been told this would happen. This was recommended practice and would give my brain time to heal.

It had been explained to Trevor that I would be hooked up to numerous machines and that I would be constantly monitored. I would have a nurse allocated to me and she would be with me at all times. (Although there were male nurses, I didn't have any at this time). There was also a back-up system so that if anything went amiss, alarms would go off and other staff would be there as well.

Although it can be scary to see someone in this state, Trevor was aware of what to expect, so when he finally saw me the next morning, it didn't come as a great shock.

The plan was to have me in this induced coma for 36 hours and, depending on my vital signs and how I responded, they would then intubate me and bring me out of it.

Meanwhile, back in Australia, Kristy and Steven (my children) were doing it tough. Sometimes imagination can run wild, and try as you might, negative thoughts can run amok. I'm told they didn't get much sleep and when they got the call from Trevor in the early morning hours (their time) to say that the operation was a success and I was now back in ICU, it was like they'd been holding their breath for hours.

They were so relieved.

They had asked him to phone as soon as he heard anything and naturally, they were thrilled to hear his voice. Mostly though, they were glad to hear the relief in his voice.

Tristan and Bronwyn and their spouses had also had me in their thoughts and although not related by blood, we had become so much closer because of all we'd gone through... together. They too had been anxiously awaiting good news about me.

Everyone we loved had been there for us and although the grandkids were not fully aware of the severity of the situation, we know we were constantly in their prayers.

Trevor came to see me the following morning and even though he'd been prepared, he was still shocked to see me lying there motionless. I sounded like Darth Vader as the machine I was hooked up to breathed for me.

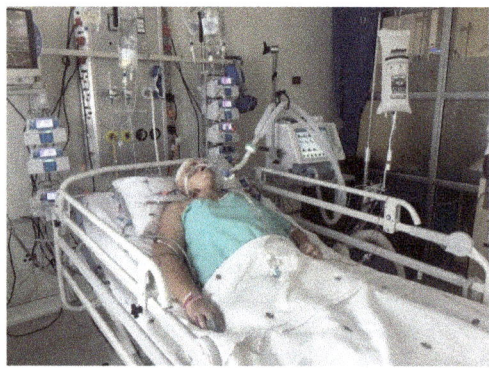

He chatted to me, held my hand and kissed me gently, not knowing what I might be aware of, if anything. He spent most of the day by my bedside keeping vigil while the nurses attended to my every need.

Along with the news that the operation was successful was the even better news that Dr. Timakia had managed to get **all** of the tumour and that the frozen section showed it was indeed a meningioma, as Tristan, Trevor's son had suggested, and – the best news of all – that it was benign.

Dr. Timakia said the post-operative period might be protracted but the fact I had a potentially very curative tumour was extremely reassuring. He was hopeful that I would be woken the next day (Wednesday), as was planned, and that he thought there would be no need for chemotherapy, but I would need to have follow-up MRI brain scans for several years to come, just to ensure it did not grow back.

Wow …all of that wonderful news in one hit!

Trevor immediately relayed all of this to our family and there was a real sense of joy on hearing this, even though they all knew I wasn't out of the woods yet.

There was still a huge risk of infection. My brain could swell causing encephalitis and I was also very susceptible to having a seizure.

No one knew yet whether I would be back to my old self, with all my senses fully intact (the best scenario we could hope for), or whether the way I was before the operation would end up being as good as I got, or if there would be a slow recovery which hopefully saw me back to being close to my old self, or close enough to it or whether I'd sustained further brain damage.

We all knew that even given the best scenario, recovery could take a long time. It would probably be 18 months before I would have my full brain function back.

Angelique, the ambulance attendant who'd brought me to the hospital in the first place, had been a constant visitor. She came to see me early in the morning the day after my surgery to find me vitally stable and in an induced coma. She stood by the door of my room and said a short prayer for me and when she came back later in the day and saw Trevor sitting in a chair, reading, she was so glad he'd been allowed to stay close to me all that time.

He stayed with me for most of the time I was in my induced coma, even though I have no memory of this.

So much had happened in a mere week!
I'd been taken off the ship.
I'd had an MRI brain scan.
I'd been told I had a huge brain tumour.
I'd been admitted to intensive care.
I'd had a craniotomy and had my meningioma removed.
I'd been put in an induced coma.

These were just the facts, the things that happened. Each of these came with their own set of emotions and each of these things impacted Trevor and me in very different ways.

Whilst all of this was happening to me, it was so much worse for Trevor, because he was the one who had taken the brunt of most of it.

In hospital I had everything done for me; he was the one who had attended to everything and made all the decisions and kept everyone informed. If given the choice, I know I had the best end of the deal.

I think he said it so well when he described how the last week had made him feel like 'a piece of chewed string'. It had been such a stressful week for us, but especially for him.

We knew though, that no matter what came after, our lives had been changed forever and as strange as it may sound, we both knew without a doubt, that it was very much for the better and we would both be better people because of it.

We never once said: 'Why us?'

We knew that this experience was a test, a challenge and a gift, all in one.

We had met so many really lovely people over that week; people who took the time to come and visit and we had made lasting friendships as a result.

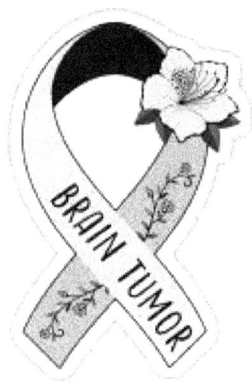

The journey within is a journey of the heart,

And there is no right or wrong way to get

there.

When you get there, feel the completeness

And contentment within that allows

Your mind to rest and accept love.

Love is your way to peace

And peace is your way to love.

The two may be separate

But one cannot be without the other.

CHAPTER 15

From Tuesday, February 25

People often wonder what happens when you're in a coma. I was certainly asked this on lots of occasions.

'Did I see a tunnel or a white light? If not that, what did I see? What did I feel? What did I experience?'

I know that usually when you are in an operating theatre, you are asked to count backwards from 10 and before you get to the magic number of zero, you're out cold. I suppose they didn't ask me to do that because of my inability to talk.

I was no sooner settled in the theatre and I was out like a light. I felt nothing, I heard nothing, but I experienced lots of things.

Some might say I dreamt it, but I know better.

There are dreams where you wake up remembering what happened in them and you can recall every single event in great detail. Some are just so crazy you wonder how your brain actually conceptualised them.

There are others that leave you frightened and, even though you know they weren't real, the feeling stays with you for a long time.

There are some that just flit through your subconscious mind and leave clues for your consciousness to take up if it so chooses and there are so many that are just our brain defragging itself from the daily rigours of life, most of which we do not even remember.

For me, time stood still, or should I say, there was no such thing as time. I was in this beautiful place that had no bounds; that had no shape, colour or form and there, right in front of me, were my mum and my dad.

My Mum and Dad.

It was like they were with me the entire time. Although I could only see them from their hips up, I had the feeling they were standing, and although they weren't holding hands as they used to do so often, they were standing side-by-side, shoulder to shoulder, looking at me as one unit. They were wearing soft pastel colours, and even though I couldn't describe the colours, or what they wore, it added to the aura of gentleness and love they exuded.

It was like nothing else existed except for the three of us — them and me. I felt I couldn't take my eyes off them and neither did I want to. I felt that they had come to me together as one unit, giving me strength to get through this.

They didn't say a word; they didn't smile as such, but both their faces were gentle, soft and beautiful.

I couldn't touch them because I knew they were out of reach. I wanted for nothing and I asked for nothing.

The peace I felt was like something I've rarely experienced before, and I knew without a doubt they had been there for me in spirit, in my hour of need.

On an inner level, I felt strong, and I knew I would get through this, even if it was going to take some time.

I wasn't going to let my Mum and Dad down. They were expecting me to be my very best and that's what I would give with this new chance.

On the morning of February 26, I was intubated and thankfully I have no recollection of this procedure. I believe it's not the most pleasant experience, but all went well, and I woke.

Hans and Rowena, my brother and sister-in-law were driving from Durban to Richards Bay to see us later in the day. The ship had docked there and instead of going on a tour like they had originally planned, they wanted to be with us. Trevor had contacted them and let them know I'd had the operation and it had gone well.

Knowing they were coming, I think I willed myself to be awake and well enough for them.

They were to arrive at midday on the Wednesday and my induced coma had commenced Monday about 9pm – it would be cutting it fine.

But I made it!

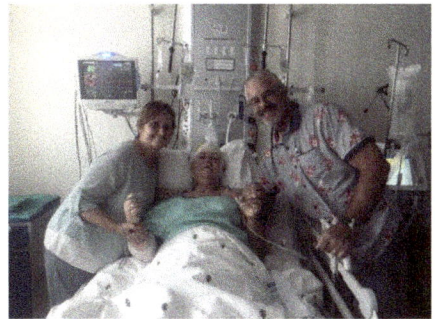

Waking up with Hans and Rowena at my side.

Seeing them both and seeing the concern on their faces really humbled me.

I knew they'd gone to a lot of effort to do this and be there for both of us. I think in some ways they needed to do it for themselves as well. They needed to see for themselves that I was okay.

In the past week, a lot had happened for them as well. They had been through a similar, albeit mini-rollercoaster to what we'd been through, not knowing exactly what the outcome would be. Unlike our family and friends though, they had been with us both when Fred had first started to make his presence known and they were with us both throughout the swift progression of these symptoms. They also had the advantage of knowing firsthand, the area we were in, having been there on February 17 when we'd arrived and knowing it wasn't as primitive as so many people think.

I felt such joy when Trevor said to me: 'Look who's here to visit you.'

If I could have, I would have rushed to them and hugged them so tightly, but I felt so weak, I could barely raise my head.

Hans went to my left side and Rowena to my right, and they held my hands and spoke gently to me. They had bought me a red wire hippopotamus and they said it was symbolic. Much later when I read up on the full meanings and symbolism, I realised what a wonderful gift this was for me – something to remind me always that, just like the hippo, I was born great and that I have the potential to become whoever I want to be.

I have always loved symbols of things. I practiced doing Dream/Vision Boards regularly and used to teach people how to do these. I have always had pictures on my own Dream/Vision Board that depicted what I wanted, what I wanted to become and what I wanted to have in my life. I also had ornaments in clear sight around my house as constant reminders of these as well. So, this hippopotamus was the most perfect gift for me, and the symbolism was perfect as well.

It symbolised hope, not in the usual sense, but hope in the sense that nothing is permanent in this world, something we had both come to realise all too well.

It was also about the use of aggression in the right context and how we all need to find and use our hidden strengths to influence and get the best outcomes.

A hippopotamus is a great symbol of strength and courage, calmness during crisis, maternal instincts and the ability to navigate through emotions with clarity as well as recognising the creative gifts you possess and letting these revitalise you and make you feel alive again.

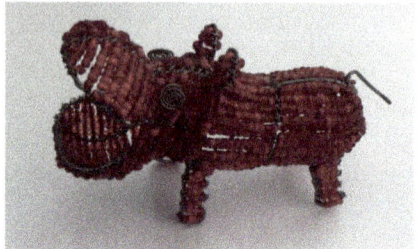

My hippopotamus gift.

In the few years prior to my tumour being discovered I had certainly lost my creativity and now that Fred was gone, it was time to bring all that creativity and intuition back to life, whilst living a well-grounded, balanced and practical lifestyle.

The other gift they gave me was a really beautifully written, sensitive novel, *Where The Crawdad Sings*. Although I was in no state to read it then, it is one of those special books that has a place in my library at home as well as in my heart.

I thought when Hans gave it to me, that it must be a text of some kind. I had asked him to research books and information I could use to retrain my brain. I had heard so much about neuroplasticity and wanted a simple guide or text, so imagine my surprise, and subsequent delight when I realised that this was his choice for me – something that filled my senses with pleasure and joy.

Hans and Rowena were only able to stay for a short period and were very aware of my frail condition. They were so pleased though, that even just out of my coma, I was thinking clearer and the few words I said were coming out fluently. They knew that the doctor's skill was unsurpassed and that my strength, courage, faith and determination would do the rest. They could leave now, knowing I was safe and in the best place possible.

They said their goodbyes and as I leaned forward, so did the contents of my stomach. Thank goodness Rowena had lots of experience in nursing and wasn't particularly perturbed with catching the contents (the lengths love will go to). A nurse was soon on hand though and scurried them out of the room while she cleaned me up. When they came back, I said goodbye again.

I was very aware of the importance of having lots of time up your sleeve to get back to the ship just in case anything should go wrong and the ship sails without you. I was therefore doubly grateful that, although it had only been a relatively short visit, they'd taken so much time and made so much effort for me.

Trevor took them out for lunch and even though we'd both met really wonderful people, being with Hans and Rowena again was like slipping on a familiar, well-worn slipper. It was so comfortable and there was no hesitancy whatsoever in what was talked about. Trevor had a real laugh with them when they relayed their dramas about getting a rental car.

When on the ships, the passengers are constantly warned about pickpockets and being taken advantage of by some of the locals. This is not done in a derogatory manner, just as a precautionary warning so passengers being in a strange land do not take unnecessary risks.

Because their trip to visit me was a last-minute thing, all the rental cars from all the reputable companies had already been booked. Passengers and locals had done this well in advance to ensure they could go on safaris. When it came to Hans and Rowena trying to get a car at this last minute, the only dealer they could find was one with a residential (not business) address on the outskirts of town.

'A bit dodgy', they thought.

The owner of the company asked them to come to his home and they could discuss the terms there. Alarm bells began ringing.

Hans told me later that he and Rowena had lots of concerns over it, but in the end, they knew it was the only way they could see me, so very hesitantly, they agreed.

When they got there, they were met by his wife and felt very silly to see all their initial concerns were unfounded. They were a really charming couple who bent over backwards to help them.

In fact, so many things went in their favour.

They got a fabulous, latest-model Mercedes-Benz sports car. It was so luxurious and had so many gadgets, they were afraid to press any buttons that weren't explicitly labelled in case they did something wrong.

Their visit, wonderful though it was, made me very tired and over the next few days I slept a lot. I can now understand why visiting times are limited and I also understand why Trevor was allowed to be with me for such extended periods. He never drained my energy. If I wanted or needed to sleep, he would just pick up his book and read it. I'm sure if the staff had noticed that he was draining my energy, they would have asked him to leave. As it was, he was a real tonic for me, better than any medicine they could give me.

I'm sure I was still on a number of drugs after I was awoken and although I did experience a lot of discomfort from the shunts and tubes lodged at the back of my head, making it difficult to put my head in a comfortable position, I did not need and did not want any analgesics.

The evening after I was intubated, the drains they'd put into the back of my head to stop any buildup of fluid and prevent risk of infection were removed and the sites were sutured shut. This was another step forward.

The nurses were just wonderful during this initial phase. I was totally bedridden, and they bathed me and looked after all my physical needs.

People can often feel very vulnerable having everything done for them but in my case, I knew I couldn't do much at all for myself, so there really was no choice.

I remember reading a beautiful book called *Tuesdays With Morrie* by Mitch Albom. It was about a man who suffered ALS (Lou Gehrig's disease). It was based on a true story and if you haven't read it, I would highly recommend it.

As Morrie's situation deteriorates to the point where he is totally dependent on others to attend to all his physical needs, he becomes very grateful for the kind acts everyone bestows upon him. Rather than being upset by the situation and the degradation of the position he is in, he feels gratitude for those around him. Although I was only in this position for a short period of time, I thought to myself: 'I'll do a Morrie' and so I offered each of these experiences up as a prayer of gratitude.

Each and every one of the nurses was wonderful and there were a few that I became especially close to (I'm sure they know who they are). My gratitude to them knows no bounds.

During this time my brain was like a computer that had been turned off and now needed to reboot itself. I had very limited thought and I found I could only concentrate on one thing at a time and then only for a very limited time.

I was very tired a lot of the time and did what was best for my brain; I slept a lot.

When Angelique took a detour via my room and saw me awake, she was surprised that I looked so much more alert than when they'd first picked me up just over a week before from the ship.

She continued to visit me almost daily and told me later what a privilege it had been seeing me progress and allowing her to have this unique learning opportunity as she walked with me on my path to healing.

Obviously, there was still a long way to go in my recuperation before I would be ready to take the long flight home but at this stage, if all went well, it looked like it would be another three weeks or so.

When Trevor sent his regular emails to people we knew around the globe, he consistently commented on my courage and acceptance of the situation. As far as I was concerned, though, I was so very lucky and when you've been blessed this way, you only have gratitude in your heart. I knew without a doubt as well, that the universe was certainly on our side. How could we doubt it with all the coincidences we had experienced?

As if Princess Cruises hadn't already done enough for us, they had almost daily contact with Trevor or both of us to ensure they were doing and supporting us as best they could. Meanwhile they were still trying to sort out what was happening with Trevor's next cruise on the Pacific Princess, a world cruise he was due to board from The Maldives.

Because I'd gotten through the operation and was now in the recovery phase, he would be leaving within the week and hopefully Kristy, my daughter would be coming over. We still weren't sure if the insurance company would cover her costs, but we were hopeful. She would have to pay for her return tickets up front and then if Cover-More Travel Insurance agreed, they would reimburse her. It was a risk, but she was insistent she was coming over, even if they weren't agreeable.

Up until this point, Trevor had really only seen the environs of the hospital when we first arrived, the countryside to and from the hospital to the Indaba Lodge and the mall near the hospital. However, now he knew I was on my road to recovery, he thought he'd do a bit more exploring of the area and perhaps even go on a safari in the week prior to him going on the next cruise. The days were long, and he could fit this in either prior to seeing me or afterwards. I was so excited for him to do this and although I would have loved to have been by his side and enjoyed it with him, it was more important to me that he didn't miss this opportunity a second time, especially seeing we were right at the gates of the most renowned African national parks in the world.

To be able to do this, he was hopeful that Princess Cruises would look into hiring a car for him rather than providing the taxi service. It would possibly be a much cheaper option for them and definitely a lot less restrictive for Trevor. However, the taxi service continued, and Trevor was very mindful not to abuse the privilege and only used it to go to the hospital and return from the hospital back to the lodge.

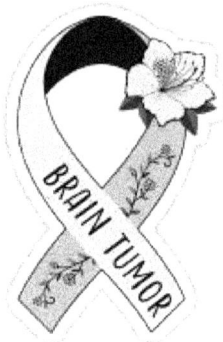

Be brave for you are yet to meet
Your true challenge and destiny.

Feel the ripples of excitement
As you come into yourself
And learn the true depths of your soul.

Release all that is superfluous
And all that is no longer needed
And weighs you down.

You find true peace not through doing
But through being your true self.

CHAPTER 16

Thursday and Friday, February 27 and 28

I had some very interesting, frightening and also disturbing thoughts and experiences over the next few days after I was taken out of my comatose state, and these led to a few very profound decisions I made for my future life.

I was in a semi-conscious state on and off, drifting in and out of sleep and my other fantasy, nightmarish world.

Although my bed in the ICU was the same one that I'd had since I was first admitted there and the room was the same, I believed I was somewhere else and that, rather than lying flat, I was actually lying in an upright position a lot of the time. This was a really weird sensation and one I found difficult to get my head around. How could I be lying upright and why?

My mattress was designed with air pockets that would inflate and then deflate, reducing the risk of pressure areas. There were also Velcro cuffs on my ankles that did the same thing, like the cuff on a blood pressure machine. The mattress and cuffs around my ankles automatically inflated and deflated in a rhythmical pattern several times an hour. These were utilised while I was in my coma as well as several days after this.

In my semi-conscious state, my world closed in on me and I could make no sense of anything that was happening around me. All I saw was blackness all around me and each time the air mattress deflated, I felt like I was being sucked into a dark hole I could not escape from, deep into its blackness it kept sucking me in!

This was one of the most frightening experiences I have ever had in my life.

I was powerless physically as I was sucked deeper and deeper into its hold. I couldn't move. I couldn't even open my eyes. I tried to call for help but I knew that nobody could hear me.

I felt like this was the end for me and I was terrified.

My body felt like my buttocks were in the middle of a large circular ring (like one of those plastic swimming rings you use in a pool) and it was being sucked down deeper and deeper and the rest of my body was being sucked down, down, down into it – deeper and deeper until I felt I couldn't breathe.

Everything around me was black; everything was dark; it felt to me like hopelessness.

What could I do when I was totally powerless and helpless?

And then the answer came and certainly not in the way I would have expected.

My thoughts went to all those poor people who are in the last stages of cancer where there really is no hope and no escape from the pain and suffering ahead of them and I felt a deep compassion for them. I couldn't imagine what it must be like to stare into this abyss for months on end with nothing but suffering, pain and indescribable loss ahead of you.

It was like I was being shown how things could have gone. I could have been in a world that was filled with darkness and despair, with no voice and a total dependence upon others to do for me the things I could no longer do for myself, due the loss of my physical strength and co-ordination.

On another level though, this highlighted to me the way I'd always played it small. I'd often been scared of taking chances because I didn't believe in my strengths and abilities.

This was a pivotal moment in my life, and I knew that the choice I made at this stage would determine the rest of my life.

This was the first lesson I learned.

I would will myself to get well – no matter what it took – and I would appreciate and give my best and do my best with every moment of my life. I would appreciate every gift I had and feel proud to share each of them.

Amazingly, as soon as I came to this decision, the fear and feelings left me and I slumbered peacefully, awaking with the memory of what I'd gone through as well as the powerful lesson I'd learned.

Next time in my semi-conscious state, when my brain started to fire again, I became aware of lots of colours.

Whenever I had meditated in the past, I would usually see a beautiful magenta colour. This would indicate to me that I was in the zone.

However, the colours I saw during this time were very different. I saw shades of bright red flowing through my veins and arteries spreading vitality around my entire body and then I saw a murky blue/green colour in my head. It was as if these colours were cleaning up the remaining debris in my brain. I felt that although Fred was completely gone, my brain just needed that final mop-up.

I could actually visualise these colours going into all the little nooks and crannies that the surgeon's instruments might have failed to reach. It was like I had been cleansed entirely by colour and this reassured me on a much deeper, spiritual level.

On Thursday morning, three days after surgery and the day after awaking from my coma, Dr. Lucelle came to see me. It was about 7.30am and I'd already been awake for a number of hours. I was so relieved to see her and as my emotions got the better of me, I just burst into tears. I knew that this was actually a healthy release of my emotions and certainly not a histrionic display. However, every time I'd cried previously, the nurses had been very concerned because it raised my blood pressure.

Dr. Lucelle told me it was a very natural thing to do, and rather than stop me crying, she let me talk. I loved her for this. I did understand the concern the nurses had, but I've always believed that emotions are better out than in, and after all I'd been through, I knew I needed this release valve.

When Kristy, my daughter, was six years old, after her father and I had divorced, I had bought her a book that helped explain the feelings that could often arise in children when their parents divorce. I'll never forget some of the wisest words I ever heard:

'You've got to let the bad feelings out, so that the good feelings can grow.'

I talked to Dr. Lucelle about my concerns about being such a burden to Trevor and I wondered what he would be really thinking of me with my bald head, and would he still love me?

It was so nice to express these thoughts to a woman, especially someone I trusted implicitly and felt such an affinity with. I didn't feel judged, and she normalised all I was feeling and never once said I was being silly. In fact, although she said she was sure my concerns were unfounded, she agreed that I should feel free to express myself and that crying was probably the best medicine for me. So as one of my doctors, she prescribed a good cry!

This was the second lesson I learnt:

Never be afraid to express my emotions. I own them and it doesn't matter what anyone else thinks or says about them – they are mine and are valid to me.

When Trevor arrived an hour or so later, I was still a bit teary. I felt really fragile and without saying anything, he just came over to me and gently held me in his arms. He stroked my face being careful not to hurt me and asked me what was wrong.

'I'm so sorry I've got no hair now and I must look so ugly to you. How could you love me like this?' I blubbered into his shoulder.

He told me I would always be beautiful to him and that nothing could change the way he felt about me. He loved me for the person I was, and he couldn't be prouder of me. He also said I had a really nice-shaped head and I looked great with my new 'Sinead O'Connor hairstyle'.

He was so real and as usual, he could make me laugh, even if it was at myself.

It was strange for me to have been so concerned about my hair (or lack of it) at this time for various reasons. People who know me well, know that I like my hair to look good and that I tend to travel with enough products to achieve this. However, when I was asked prior to the operation if I wanted my hair partly shaved or completely shaved, I immediately chose to have it completely shaved off. I really wasn't upset at the fact that I would be bald (something that really surprised me at the time). Trevor and I both knew that my hair would be all gone, so it was no surprise to Trevor. In fact, just before my surgery, he cut a piece of my hair (my cowlick) and had put a rubber band around it and put it in his wallet as a keepsake.

The other thing, was, that he'd seen me several times already – in my coma and after I'd woken from it – and he'd never been any different towards me because I didn't have hair. I realised how silly I'd been to have these insecure feelings, but I also knew I was human, and it was quite likely these would arise again in the future.

There was a very special nurse, Gugu Khumala who looked after me through some of my darkest days, and something really clicked between us. I felt a very close spiritual affinity that is hard to explain and, although extremely professional, I believe she felt this as well.

In one of my less lucid moments, I believed there was a specific process that would make tablets easier to swallow. I have always had a lot of difficulty swallowing tablets and have a real fear of choking.
Several years ago, Trevor had bought me these beautiful teardrop earrings. They were handmade and the design was created using silk thread.

My belief (at this time) was that if you put the tablets through this (the threads), then it would make them easier to swallow. Imagine my distress when I tried to tell Sister Khumala that this was all she had to do. Then imagine my further distress when she just didn't understand!

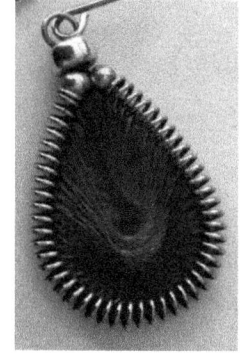

I mean, it wasn't very nice of her to make it hard on me when if she'd just followed this simple process, those little suckers would slip right down with no problem at all.

She just kept trying (very patiently) to coax me while I very stubbornly refused. In the end though, she won.

It's amazing the tricks the mind can play on us and how it can determine the way we behave.

I started to develop considerably more strength in my body, and it was decided to remove my catheter. This meant that I would now be able to go to the toilet. At this stage I was still hooked up to my monitoring equipment so I would need to use the call button and have the nurse assist me.

When I slept, I slept really deeply and in early hours of the Friday morning, I awoke and I really needed to go to the toilet to relieve my bladder. In my semi-conscious state I thought I'd been told not to bother anyone so I just lay there, scared to call out, because I'd been told not to!

My mind was really groggy and my thoughts were not rational. If they had been, of course I would have rung the buzzer. Instead, I continued to lie there whilst my bladder continued to swell to the point that I thought to myself: 'I'm going to wet the bed!'

I would have been devastated if I did this. I know the nurses would have taken it in their stride, but I would have felt really ashamed and embarrassed. So, in this moment I learned my third lesson:

Never be afraid to ask for what you want. You may not get it, but if you don't even ask, you don't even give anyone the opportunity to say yes, no or maybe.

So, I pressed the call button and of course no one had said that I couldn't call them. Imagine my relief on several counts ... aaaggghhh!

These were very important lessons for me because as I was growing up, I'd been taught certain things:
- Respect your elders.

- Speak only when spoken to and never offer an opinion unless you're expressly asked to do so.
- Ask for permission to do, speak or act and wait until permission is given.
- Suppress your feelings and don't express them.
- God is always watching you, so be good at all times.
- Don't be loud or boisterous.
- If you want to play, play outside.
- Play is on the condition that all of your chores are done first.
- You can't have fun and joke around if anyone else is unhappy.
- Hugs and cuddles are for small children.
- You shouldn't say I love you too often because it loses its meaning.
- If anything goes wrong, it's likely you did something that triggered it.
- If there is conflict around you, you need to find a way to fix it.

Now in themselves some of these are very good basic rules to help guide, direct and set limits on your child in order that they grow up with basic good values.

The problem for me was that they continued as I grew older as well, and with someone with my personality, who wanted to please and not rock the boat for fear of tension in the household (which had huge consequences to my mother and brothers), I then started to self-enforce these as well. Later in my life there were a lot of experiences that reinforced these even more.

This was why I believe I was given these major lessons and I know they are now a big part of me.

My early upbringing and the lessons I learned then, provided me with a guide to good behaviour. However, I saw it as a rule book, rather than a guidebook. There were a lot of things I should have challenged, and if I had done so, I know my life would have had a lot more joy and love in it.

Throughout most of my life, I'd waited for people to give me permission and I'd battled with feelings of unworthiness. I'd felt uncomfortable asking for anything for myself and when it came to expressing my feelings, I often believed they were either wrong, or weren't validated.

This chance at a new life was my chance to do things differently.

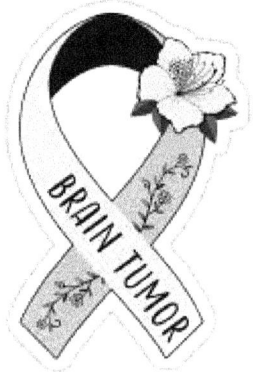

What may appear as errant thoughts
Are also not random.

They are specks and stars upon the canvas
That becomes the tapestry of 'you'.

It is 'You' who chooses each thought
To be either a fleeting one
Or one you harness
As a concept or belief that you
Develop into your Mantra.

It is 'You' who chooses the path you take
And decides the 'when', the 'where'
And the 'how'.

CHAPTER 17

Mentally I was still limited to one definite thought at a time, so I had to choose wisely. I decided now Fred was gone, I would only fill my brain with positive thoughts because I knew that if I did that, a positive, happy life would be sure to follow.

I found I had to try to hang on to each of my thoughts, because if I didn't, they would escape, and I would find it difficult to get them back. I had to be really disciplined, taking each thought and developing it through to its fruition so it would not flutter away into the ether.

As before, I remained totally cognisant of all that was going on around me, only now I was able to engage and interact much better in conversations. I didn't stumble over my responses the way I had before, and although I was still not up to *reading, writing and'rithmatic*, the improvement in me was profound and really promising.

My difficulty was with the production of new thoughts and the development of these.

In my quiet times when I had nothing but the television and my thoughts, there were three basic things that I became really focused on, to the point where I could think of nothing else.

I became concerned about our finances and I tried to work out how we would survive now that I wouldn't be able to work. After all, we would be down to one income now and we still had a mortgage to pay. I kept trying to come up with all sorts of ways I could help out. I knew that the best scenario would be that I would not be fit for work for a minimum of six months, but the most likely scenario was that we were looking at an 18-month period, if not longer. Worst-case scenario would be that work as I knew it as a nurse would no longer be an option for me, ever.

Fortunately though, my mind had returned to its naïve state where nothing seemed impossible. I was so filled with this feeling of hope and promise that I was determined to have nothing stand in my way.

Naturally, my thoughts were quite unrealistic at this time, because I didn't have the ability yet to think laterally. Also, my concrete thinking meant I was unable to factor in and take into account other variables.

I had been using a wonderful nutrition program for about five years and I attributed my good health, even though I'd had a brain tumour, to this program. At my age, I was on no other medications, my vital signs had remained stable throughout my admission and I'd always been reasonably fit and able-bodied.

I knew it was time to do this program (properly) again. Although I'd continued to use a lot of the products, I had become a little bit complacent, and I'd stopped cleansing my body. I realised that investing in my health is the biggest, best investment I could make, and I was going to reinvest in me. This was indeed a very rational decision and would certainly be of great benefit in all aspects of my life.

However, up to that date, I had already created a small but steady residual income from it as well and my next thought was to re-contact with my dear friend and upline and ask her to help me get the business side back on track. At that stage I thought I just had to click my fingers and it would all magically happen. I'd forgotten the amount of hard work and dedication this would take on my part to really develop this as a long-term business (rewarding as it is).

With regard to feeding my brain with everything positive, other than doing this program, I figured it was time to get a personal success mentor. I had been following Brendon Burchard for a number of years and loved his philosophies. Everything he said made so much sense to me.

In my unrealistic state of mind, I thought it would be totally reasonable to contact him personally, tell him of my situation and ask him to train my brain from the beginning – like an experiment that could benefit both of us. I would give him access to this blank slate of a brain of mine, and he could then imprint success on my brain – easy peasy!

Naturally, this was entirely impractical, unreasonable and certainly not feasible. Over time, I have continued to enjoy his podcasts and books and find they add value to my life.

I still would love to have been his special project though because part of me still wonders if this could have made for an interesting, positive experiment.

This period of mental belief that everything was possible lasted for a few days before I came back to the land of reality. I certainly didn't come back with a thud, because for me, life is about looking at the positive in any situation and looking at the personal strengths I have to overcome any setback either from within myself or from outside of myself.

This experience highlighted to me how easy it is to have my bubble burst and how easily my positive demeanour could once again be filled with anxiety, doubt, fear and uncertainty. I also realised how vigorously I had to work on myself to keep myself positive and avoid being complacent.

I had always been aware of the importance of living a balanced life and this concept became even more important to me.

In the past I'd divided each day into four categories – mental, physical, emotional and spiritual. At the end of each day, I would then reflect on my day and if I couldn't put a tick in each of those columns indicating I'd done something fulfilling in each of those areas of my life, I knew I was in trouble and that my life was going into a downhill spiral. I knew this was a very easy and practical accountability strategy for me to continue. To this day it is my accountability tool for myself.

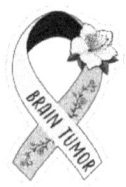

Illuminate your mind

And open your heart.

Be warm and steadfast,

Be kind and gracious,

Be discerning and loyal,

Be well tempered and restrained,

Be cautious and trusting,

Be loving and dignified.

If you are all of these things

You will shine and your light

Will fill the darkness in others.

CHAPTER 18

It's amazing, even to me, how quickly I recovered. A lot of this was due to the encouragement and support of the wonderful team I had with me – my family, my friends, Dr. Timakia, Dr. Lucelle, the wonderful nurses and physiotherapists and my special new friends, Sharmilla, Angelique and Tamsin.

I had no idea that my life was going to be even more enriched.

Dr. Lucelle came to see me, and looking at the most amazing improvement in me, she asked if both Trevor and I would like to join her and her family at the church they go to on the following day.

What! Go out?

That sounded amazing and so, with the blessing of Dr. Timakia and the entire ICU staff, we went off to church the following day.

I had asked Dr. Lucelle to bring me in a scarf to cover my head (more to avoid any risk of infection rather than embarrassment) and she brought in a lovely choice of which I thought the one with tigers was the most apt (considering where we were).

I remember going down the lift in a wheelchair and then meeting her beautiful family – Kenneth, her husband and Michael and Gabriel her twin boys. It was a bit tricky for me negotiating the step down from the kerb and then the step up into the car, but with so many hands giving me assistance, I managed it well.

We drove about 15 minutes and this time I saw the countryside properly, not as I'd done before from the back of an ambulance. It was really green and reminded me of home.

We got to the church and I knew that if I didn't feel well, I could go back to the hospital at any time. Although I was still really weak, I felt good within myself. I was happy and I loved being outside away from the confines of hospital. I was not going to miss out on this experience for love nor money.

On arrival, Dr. Lucelle introduced us to Pastor Cecil Pillay, who welcomed us like we were friends he'd just never met before. We later found out that it was very unusual for her to invite anyone to church with her, so this was indeed something very special she did for us.

The atmosphere in this church was indescribable. There was music, singing, coloured lights and the thread that held it all together was the love and wise words that emanated from

Pastor Cecil. His sermon was an inspiration and when he called us to come to the front of the church, we both felt humbled and proud to be there with him, his family and this wonderful congregation who opened their hearts to us travellers. He invited Trevor to sing a few songs as well and we left this church feeling enlightened and enriched deep into our souls.

We still remember Pastor Cecil's wise, prophetic words: '2020, a year of plenty, plenty.'

Over the past few months, we'd certainly already experienced plenty of drought, bushfires and floods and the new year had barely begun. However, I'm sure he didn't mean it in a negative context. We just had a quiet chuckle to ourselves and often when we think of 2020, we are reminded of his words and smile as we think of him.

After church we went to a hotel and were treated to lunch by Dr. Lucelle and Kenneth (or should I say, a banquet).

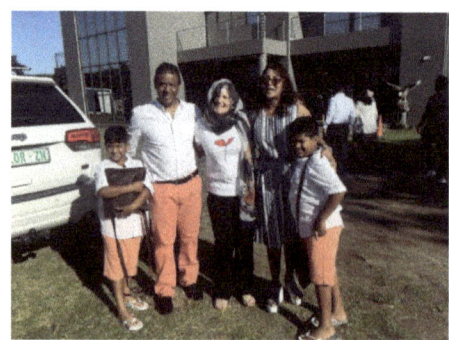

My first outing.

The authentic African food was absolutely delicious and as we ate by the shoreline, we all got to know each other better and realised, although we live thousands of miles apart, we had so much in common on so many levels.

Their two boys were such a delight and, although twins, were as different as chalk and cheese, both in looks and behavior. We laughed at the antics of the monkeys, something we don't get to see in Australia, and were warned not to encourage them in any way, shape or form.

Dr. Lucelle, Kenneth and the boys couldn't get enough of Trevor's stories and we all laughed and talked for hours. It was such a tonic for me.

When it was time to go back to the hospital, although I was ready to do so after such a big day, I did so with the knowledge we had added so many more people to our growing list of lifelong friends.

The following day Trevor came in with a wonderful surprise for me. He'd brought in his guitar and sang to me.

He doesn't always sing the songs I love to hear, but he indulged me with all of my favourites, as well as the songs that have become very special for both of us.

He took me on this wonderful emotional rollercoaster of our lives together and in that moment, my love for him just overflowed and as I felt the tears rolling down my face. I know he felt it too because I could hear the emotion in his voice.

I was once again in awe of this wonderful man who seventeen years ago had vowed to be with me through the good and bad times, in sickness and in health, through richer or poorer. He had kept every one of his promises and I knew without a doubt, as my mother had said to me not long before we got married, that *'this was the man for me!'*

When the nurses heard him singing, they made an excuse to just drop by and were really keen to hear more of him. Kenneth was going to try to organise an impromptu concert at either one of the hospital's function rooms or at the local golf resort.

Later that afternoon, we saw Dr. Timakia in his office, and he told us both he was pretty certain I would make a full recovery with no loss of brain or physical functioning.

It was obvious how resilient and determined I was, and that with so much to live for, that's exactly what I would be doing, living life to the fullest.

On the practical side, he did say it would still be a couple of weeks before I would be ready to return to Australia. A medic would probably need to be organised to fly with me in case I had a seizure or needed medical attention.

We also discussed that Kristy would be coming over some time before March 13 (when Trevor would be off on his world cruise) and we were very keen for him to meet her. One of the reasons for this was so she could be made familiar with my care but mostly it was so I could show her off to him. After all, I was so very proud of her and the way she'd come to the party for us.

Not blowing my own trumpet, but I know I was a favourite at the hospital and that a lot of the staff saw me as their 'miracle patient'. I was indeed one of the luckier ones there, and I knew this. I was the recipient of lots of visitors and Trevor was always a constant by my bedside. Everyone and everything around me was just so wonderful.

I felt sorry for some of the other patients because they had no visitors and some even died while I was there, alone and unloved in those final moments.

Although I was often told how brave and courageous I was, I never saw myself that way. My philosophy has always been that God never gives you more than you can deal with. I knew there was a reason this had happened to me (to us) even though I didn't know exactly what that reason was. So, as far as I was concerned, that was all I needed to know. I just prayed for the strength to deal with things whenever I started to falter.

We continued to get emails from our family overseas with lots of words of encouragement and we tried as often as we could to do Face-time with our close family. It was so great being able to talk normally and to feel so hopeful about our future.

I hadn't wanted to go down the track of what would have happened to Trevor if I'd died. I knew for a fact that it would have changed his life profoundly. After you've found a love like we shared there is nothing that could possibly compare.

Knowing this, I would not have wanted him to live the rest of his days alone and would have wanted him to experience love, however it came in his life.

I knew he would always have our children and grandchildren, but I also knew he would need more. He loves people, music, telling stories and has so much to give and I would have hated to see this be cut short if for some reason my life had ended prematurely.

I was so lucky when our lives crossed at a time when I thought I would never experience love again and I know he felt exactly the same and, although everyone faces their own mortality at some time in their lives, our doing so together really changed the way we both saw and continue to see life and love and value the things that really matter.

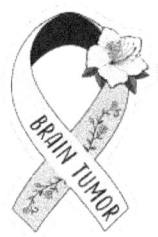

Realise that your gifts are your gifts alone.
Realise that a gift is never a gift
Until it is given to another
Or shared in unison.

Be brave for you have yet to meet
Your true challenge and destiny.

Your life has its own design
And you are the driver
On the tracks laid before you.

The train of life does not always go full speed
And there is no turning back on this train.

CHAPTER 19

Monday, March 2... One week after surgery

Today was another milestone in my recovery. Seeing firsthand how well I was doing and how much I'd improved, Dr. Lucelle and Dr. Timakia decided to move me to the orthopaedics ward.

I couldn't understand initially why I was being transferred to this ward because I thought orthopaedics covered joint operations, knee and hip replacements and the like. I didn't for one minute think this ward was where I'd end up, until it was explained to me that my operation was one on my skull. Orthopaedics was about caring for people with any operations on any bones in their body and having just had a large part of my skull operated on, it did indeed make me a genuine contender for this ward.

Duh! Of course; it all made sense now.

Dr. Lucelle pulled a few strings and got me into a private room and realising these were few and far between, I was most appreciative. Sometimes it's not what you know, but who you know!

I had a window with a view mainly of the rooftop of the hospital, but it was a view, nonetheless. I could see outside and that was what mattered. I could see if it was sunny or rainy and more often than not, a variety of birds would fly by or sit as I looked at them in awe and envied them their ability to fly.

Things were different here. The nurses were great, but I missed the nurses in ICU. It just seemed to lack the closeness I'd become accustomed to. One definite plus here was the improvement in the menu. The choices were more varied and the food, when it came, was hot. I actually looked forward to mealtimes.

I heard the nurses talking among themselves and I knew they were having an issue with one of the patients I had been in ICU with. He'd also been moved to orthopaedics due to having had a head injury. On top of this, the doctors also suspected he had some form of dementia. To complicate things even further, he was from a foreign, non-English speaking country. The nurses couldn't identify where exactly he came from and this made it really difficult for them to communicate with him. He had become very confused and required one-on-one attention. He'd been put into a shared room and his room-mate had been very upset at having to share with him. In a private hospital, patients do express their views and their entitlements more and he certainly made it known that he did not wish to share another night with this disturbed man.

The nurses weren't sure what to do. They knew I'd been allotted the private room and didn't want to take it off me, so they very reluctantly came in to ask if I would mind giving it up. Naturally, I could understand their dilemma, having been in similar situations with difficult-to-manage patients myself, so of course I agreed.

I was actually not upset at having to share a room. In fact, I looked forward to having some company during the times when Trevor or one of my other visitors weren't there. I did insist on having the bed closest to the window, though.

Having an ensuite to myself had been a real treat in my single room, and although I loved not having to share a bathroom or toilet, imagine my surprise to find there was a bath in the two-bed ward I was moved to. What a luxury.

For the life of me though, I couldn't understand the rationale behind having a bath in an orthopaedic ward. It seemed totally irrational to me. However, I wasn't going to question it. Instead, I was looking forward to luxuriating in it each day, whilst my roommates wouldn't be able to appreciate this luxury.

Each morning I would get up early, get my scant toiletries and a change of clothes together and set myself up to have my bath. I still had some issues with my co-ordination so the chair in there became a necessity for me. Although I was able to undress without any problem (as long as I held onto something for balance), I needed to sit down to put my feet into my underpants and trousers before I could stand to slip fully into them.

The first time I got into the bath was a bit of a fiasco because I really hadn't thought it through. All was fine until I had to get out of it. I had no idea on how I was going to do this. There was no way that I could just stand up from my sitting position, even if I did use the rim of the bath for support. Firstly, I didn't have the strength and secondly, I couldn't co-ordinate myself properly.

I finally managed to manoeuvre myself into a better position, rolling myself onto all fours. Then, when I was on my knees, I grabbed the side of the bath for support as I slowly and painstakingly got myself up into a standing position. After this, I clumsily got one leg out of the bath onto the floor (which was a little bit lower than the bath), before my other leg followed. I did this holding the bath and the chair as well.

I probably should have rung the call bell for some assistance really, but my independent streak wouldn't allow it. Thank goodness my pride didn't cometh before a fall.

The difficulty I had having a bath certainly didn't deter me, and over the next few days, I became more proficient at it.

I had a number of roommates during my stay here. Each person came in for either a knee or hip replacement and only stayed a few days.

I thought it was really funny when on one occasion, my 'roomie' asked for my help to mobilise. The nurses were busy elsewhere and she wanted assistance to get to and from the toilet. She had been up and about a bit prior to this and was gaining her mobility slowly. I'm sure she had no idea of the seriousness of what I'd been through. All she saw was my shaved head and a few bandages. She probably figured it was nothing compared to **her** issue and I certainly didn't choose to enlighten her.

Having had an outing the day before being transferred to this ward, I was keen for some more outings. Trevor had been going to the mall on a regular basis and word was getting around about me. In fact, I was becoming quite the celebrity in town – sort of a 'miracle lady'.

Obviously, I wasn't out of the woods yet. There was still a risk of seizures, but the recovery that was expected to take months was taking days. It was like the rate of my improvement was mimicking my previous quick rate of deterioration.

My brain functions were returning to normal and physically I was getting stronger all the time. Although I wasn't up to sprinting anywhere and I tired easily and I often still needed an arm to lean on when I went anywhere, I knew without a doubt I was on the mend.

The physiotherapists who had visited me twice a day, every day since my operation, continued to visit. They would give me physio on my back and then take me for a walk. Initially it was just a very short distance, but then as time progressed, I began walking up and down stairs as well. I was so proud of each incremental step I made towards wellness, and I could actually understand the way both mental and physical capacities need to develop and follow specific steps. You really can't walk before you crawl.

I was so lucky that I hadn't lost my capacity to a large degree in any of these areas but nonetheless, even though things returned to me very quickly, I still struggled with the various steps that made thinking and doing tasks possible.

It had only been two weeks since we'd received such terrible news with a diagnosis and prognosis that would put fear into the bravest of men. Now, here we were, filled again with hope and promise of a future that held much for us both.

It was hard to believe we had gotten through such a dark and terrible time, but we knew it had been love, trust and faith that had gotten us to where we were now.

When I looked at Trevor, I saw how much he'd changed. I saw strengths in him that I never knew existed before.

I understood the depths of his love for me and knew he loved me enough not to ever have me as a person who wasn't able to think or do for myself (after all, he'd signed a DNR form on my behalf). This must have been one of the most difficult things he would ever have been asked to do. In doing this, he had to understand exactly how serious things were, and would have had to have been prepared to let me go, rather than hold onto me. I was so very grateful to him for doing this because I would not have wanted a life I couldn't come back from.

I have always enjoyed writing and I always found this was the perfect way to express my deepest thoughts. However, along with my inability to verbally communicate, I had also lost my ability to write. This didn't come back to me until I was well and truly settled in the orthopaedic ward. I couldn't hold a pen properly and I still couldn't get my thoughts together enough to write them down.

It was such a thrill when eventually I could do this again, so I decided that each day, I would write a page or so on what had happened that day. Most days, a page was all I needed. After all, I was only up to writing facts. I couldn't extrapolate any more than that.

As I looked over my notes, I realised how filled with gratitude I was at everything I had in my life and especially how grateful I was at the very fact that I had life. My father used to always say: 'You know it's going to be a good day when your feet are above the ground and not under the ground.'

I was very aware of how limited all our lives here on Earth are, and the importance of what we do and what we give in life. I couldn't get the image of Mum and Dad being with me several days prior to this when I really needed them the most, out of my mind. They gave me the strength, love and support that I had needed to move forward.

We all need people in our lives to do this from time to time and my parents, although not always there for me when I was younger, had made quite a trek to do this for me at this time, a time when I needed them the most.

I knew without a doubt how much they had loved me and how much they had sacrificed for me, and for this I was very grateful. Not all children grow up knowing they are loved, and I had no doubt that I was. After all, they had come 'from the other side' just to be with me!

I reflected on my family and Trevor's family and the qualities each of them had. They were all so very different, but what a team we all made together.

The sight of Kristy, Steven and my grandchildren, Jaydn, Matthew, Liam and Jake all sitting on the bed in her bedroom just chatting together when we had a Face-time conversation, really warmed my heart. I realised that even though Trevor and I were 10,500 miles from them, we were actually closer than we'd ever been.

In that moment I looked back and reflected upon the sort of mother I'd been to both Kristy and Steven, and I realised how often I'd let other, unimportant things get in the way. I wished I'd done so many things differently (as most mums do), but I also know that even though I fell short at times, my love for them knew no bounds. In the end, that's the thing children need, to be loved and know they are loved unconditionally.

I felt so grateful for all this love I felt around me, this totally unconditional love.

In that moment, I vowed I would make a positive difference in the future and in the world. I knew there was no room for negative thoughts and with a positive approach in all things for the future, I knew without a doubt, that I would be serving not only me, but my life's purpose and everyone I would be associated with in the future, for the better.

This filled me with hope and so much joy for the future ahead.

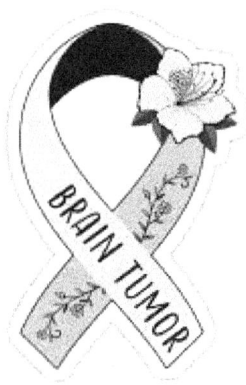

Learn your limitations,
And continue to strengthen your spirit
By being true to your convictions.

Put your trust in the master plan
Believing that the way will be made clear
for you

Negativity is the toxin of the mind.
It runs through like weeds in a garden
And can make idealism superfluous

You must constantly weed out
The negative thought patterns
Before they turn to seed.

CHAPTER 20

A life lived well is a very full life and I was determined to have more fun and do the things I really enjoyed. This is what we are supposed to do in life.

I knew today was going to be special because I'd been given permission to go to the mall. Dr. Timakia made me promise to return to the ward if I wasn't feeling well, which of course I promised him. I would have pretty much agreed to anything for a bit more of a taste of freedom.

I'm sure Trevor had no idea of what this meant to me. He'd been going to the mall regularly as part of his daily routine. He would often go over to have a cup of coffee or exchange some money or get some more phone credits while the nurses were busy attending to me. He had become quite well known to lots of the shop owners and was on first name basis with most of them.

I got up out of bed that morning feeling happy and excited. It was so nice to be wearing normal clothes as well. We left the hospital ward and, because I didn't have a scarf, my head was bare, except for the bandages that covered my huge scar. Although I wasn't self-conscious about this, I was very conscious of not leaving myself open to infection. Also, with no hair, I didn't want to have too much exposure to the sun and get a sunburned scalp. With all this in mind, my first mission was to find a scarf I could wrap around my head.

I was so lucky to find this wonderful lady in one of the shops who took the time to demonstrate the various ways I could wear it. I was so pleased with the finished result and couldn't help but sneak a glimpse of myself in the reflection of shop windows. I now fitted in with so many of the locals there who regularly wore scarves round their heads. I think this woman quite enjoyed the challenge, to be honest, and I went on my way feeling pretty chuffed with my new look.

Trevor had raved to me about the wonderful eggs benedict he'd had at a quaint little café called *The Elephant and I* and he was going to treat me to this. It was one of my favourite foods and I was salivating at the thought.

We walked up a small ramp and were shown to a table. The décor was very African with pictures and cute sculptures of elephants all around. I didn't even ask to see the menu because I knew exactly what I wanted. It was so yummy! We each had a coffee that came with two small, shortbread-style biscuits. They were to die for (figuratively speaking of course). Being a little forward, and feeling I had nothing to lose, I asked for some more, and believe it or not, every time we went in after that, we were given a few extra biscuits. We were always given such special treatment and obviously, with the service and food being so good, we went back often.

I did need to take my time though, and several times I would walk a few steps and would need to sit and rest for a short while. I knew I had to take it easy and not to expect too much from myself, but I must admit I did find this difficult. It didn't take much at all for me to feel really exhausted and, remembering my promise to Dr. Timakia, I made sure I didn't overdo it.

In one way I really did understand how miraculously far I'd come, but on the other hand I was upset at how slowly things were progressing. Given the facts of the matter and the reality of what I'd been through in such a short time, thinking these thoughts was just ludicrous.

Typically, I had Trevor's voice of reason and his reassuring words to remind me to work within my limitations and not to expect too much from myself. He never mollycoddled me, but he was always there with a hug and a helping hand if I needed it.

That afternoon we went up to see Dr. Timakia in his office. This saved him having to take extra time out of his busy schedule to go over to the hospital to see me. I suspected also that he wanted to see firsthand how I was coping out of the hospital environment. I'm sure he wanted to assess my verbal skills as well as my co-ordination and cognition.

He sat me up on his treatment table and took out a few of the staples. Although this was uncomfortable, it was nowhere near as painful as I imagined it would be.

I think he just had the most amazing healing hands and I always felt so relaxed and confident in his ability to do anything. There were more staples to come out, but he said he'd leave them for a later date.

Later that day, Trevor got word that all had been arranged for him to do an impromptu gig at the local golf club –Porky's. This was being organised for the following Sunday. It may seem strange, but I think Trevor was more excited about doing this than he'd been about doing huge concerts on board the cruise ships. Part of it was because it was all about being able to give something back. We'd been so blessed and had both been given so much. Being able to do this was just such an honour.

I was really looking forward to coming along to this as well. After all our years together, I never tire of hearing Trevor sing.

We were going to go to church as we'd done yesterday and then we would possibly have some lunch and after that we would go the golf club where Trevor would set up and do the gig.

In the meantime, Dr. Lucelle and Kenneth's two boys were really keen to learn the ukulele and Trevor was pretty keen to teach the two of them. This was organised for later in the week.

We were getting a busy schedule going.

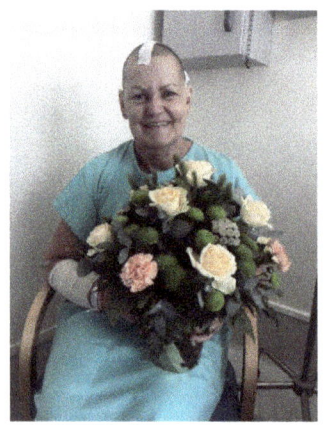

The beautiful flowers.

When I got back to the ward, I was told that the most beautiful bunch of flowers had come for me. I wasn't allowed to have flowers in intensive care, so my friends at work had waited until they were able to get them to me.

I was again awed by the love and concern from my friends and work colleagues. There had been quite a big influx of new staff over recent months and I was strangely pleased that not everyone had signed the card. In some ways it made it all the more personal to me. I don't think everyone knew what had happened to me at that stage anyway and it was on a need-to-know basis.

I was so grateful to Kristy. She'd kept all my friends from both the hospitals I worked in, informed and they knew that if they wanted any answers, they could phone her, and she would update them on my progress.

I felt so grateful for all this love and vowed I would make a positive difference in whatever small way I could in the future.

I knew there was no room for negative thoughts and with my positive approach, I knew without a doubt, that my future would entail a life of service to others. This filled me with hope and so much joy for the future ahead.

The following day, March 4, we met up with the Princess Cruises port agent, Tamsin and her mum, Brenda. What a privilege it was she had brought her mother in to meet me. We met at the hospital cafeteria and she gave us the most wonderful news – everything was now in place for Kristy to come to Richards Bay.

While the insurance company was paying for her flights, Princess Cruises were putting her up at the Indaba Lodge (where Trevor was staying) and would also be paying for all her meals. Once again, Princess Cruises were going above and beyond for us. To top it all off, they also organised for Kristy to be picked up from Durban Airport and to be driven directly to the Indaba Lodge.

My good friend, Sharmilla had also offered to pick Kristy up and take her to Indaba Lodge but we decided not to impose on her already busy schedule. There was just no end to the generosity of these strangers who were now good friends.

Sharmilla, a very private person by her own admission, told me how worried she had been for me and for both of us, especially during the long wait as I was being operated on. She said the hours had dragged for her during the period I was in my induced coma when no-one knew 'who' I would wake up to be.

I had never even considered that she would have been so worried. It just hadn't entered my head that after just meeting me only days prior to this, I had made such a huge impact upon her to make her worry so much over me. Not only was she worried, but for my sake, she believed she had to stay strong.

This was an example of the calibre of people I had with me, egging me on to get well.

Not only did I have all this emotional support and encouragement to keep my spirits up, but later that afternoon, Dr. Lucelle came in to see me with a box of my all-time favourite chocolates. I don't know how she knew they were my favourites, and I didn't ask. I just really appreciated her thoughtfulness.

Trevor wanted to bring in my mobile phone so I could phone him and he also wanted to organise for me to have a local SIM card. This posed a problem for me because I'd forgotten how to use my phone (or any mobile phone for that matter). Even though it wasn't one of the latest models, I couldn't fathom how to work out the many functions and facets. What used to be automatic for me was an impossible task. I didn't even understand how to dial a number or what buttons to press to receive a call.

On top of this, it highlighted to me that there were so many so-called simple tasks that I couldn't do any more, so I told him I didn't want my phone yet. What was the point?

The following day, Sharmilla gave me one of her old phones. This was a very basic model and one she didn't use any more.

She put a small amount of credit on it, and she spent a bit of time teaching me how to answer the phone when it rang and how to dial out on it. To simplify things for me, she also put in her and Trevor's phone numbers under favourites. That way all I had to do was look this up under contacts and press one of two buttons to reach either of them. This certainly made things very easy for me. She explained everything to me in such simple terms and she seemed to understand that my limitations were only temporary.

As the week progressed, I started to feel better and better. The physiotherapist continued to come each day and I noticed with my regular walks to the shopping centre as well as to the hospital cafeteria that I was so much better, both physically and in my general demeanour. I think it was great for Trevor not to always be in the hospital environment as well. It's not exactly the nicest place to hang out.

I felt so invigorated by rising up to the small challenges I set myself and I was reminded of the past where I'd put so many restrictions upon myself, mostly because I'd been afraid to take a chance or get out of my comfort zone. I was so excited about what my future could look like. I knew everything hinged on the choices I would make, and I was not deluding myself in thinking that everything would always be smooth sailing.

We all need ups and downs in our lives to appreciate all the variations and aspects of life. We all need challenges to get our creative thought processes going and we all need variety and stability in our lives to be able to have wings and fly.

I had been in hospital almost three weeks when Trevor asked me if I'd like to have a few hours with him at the Indaba Lodge.

'Oooh!' I thought, 'that sounds pretty good to me!'

We had not had any time totally to ourselves. There were always doctors, nurses, hospital staff and people around us, and the thought of just being alone together sounded amazing to me.

We arranged for the taxi to pick me up at the hospital and drive me to Indaba Lodge at about 9am where I would stay with Trevor for the day. I could have a sleep and we could go for a short relaxing walk and we could have a nice lunch together before I returned to the hospital late in the afternoon.

When I got there, Trevor was waiting for me and, after introducing me to the staff on duty that day, he took me up to his room.

We held each other, appreciating each other, knowing how close we had come to losing each other. He lay me down on the bed making sure that the pillows were supporting my head and not hurting it, and then he lay beside me just holding me. We fell asleep in each other's arms and when we awoke, we decided to go down to the restaurant area and order lunch.

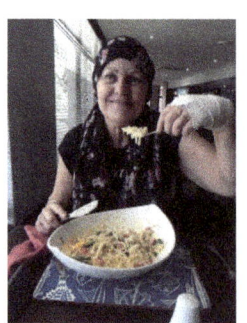

Things are a little different in certain places in South Africa and one of the big differences we noted was the amount of time it took to cook our food. There was another couple dining in the same restaurant, so it wasn't as if they were inundated. Also, we had ordered something quite basic from the menu that would have been pretty simple to put together. Well, about an hour after ordering the food, it arrived and to say it was delicious was an understatement. There was enough food on my plate to feed me for a week and it was such a shame to see it go to waste. (If I'd known, I would have asked for a half- serving).

We then had a walk around the lodge and Trevor showed me some of the wildlife and views of the bay nearby. That short walk tired me out, so we returned to his room.

I saw my suitcases on the floor and figured now was as good a time as any to rummage through them, take out what I wanted to have in the hospital with me and then pack them, so everything was organised the way I like. This time I had no difficulty doing it and it didn't take long at all. I had no need of any of my hair products, so that immediately made the job easier and I wasn't going anywhere where I needed to dress up, so all my better clothes could be packed for the trip home as well.

I got back in time for dinner but after the huge lunch I'd had, I wasn't hungry. I went to sleep early feeling really fulfilled on so many levels. What a lucky woman I was …
All that I needed now was to get back to beating Trevor at Scrabble. The only problem though was we didn't have a Scrabble board, but a trip to the mall the next day soon remedied that.

That afternoon, we sat in the hospital cafeteria and had our first post-operative game. War was declared. There was no excuse on my part anymore and Trevor wasn't going to go easy on me.

I let him win the first game, but most other games were a very close match and I really looked forward to these mental and verbal challenges. It was so good to know I hadn't lost my touch.

Usually, a cup of coffee and a piece of shared carrot cake would accompany our morning games. After all, we had to have a good reason to sit there for so long. In truth though, we were such regular customers that the staff knew us by name and were really chatty and pleasant towards us. I think they enjoyed the banter between us.

Lots of things were falling into place. Cover-More Travel Insurance continued to accept all the hospital bills and had reimbursed Trevor for all of his out-of-pocket expenses that had been incurred in the ship's medical centre and while I was in the emergency department prior to them accepting our application.

This was a weight off his mind, and it was great for him knowing his credit balance was now looking healthy again, especially knowing he would be off on another cruise.

I started using the mobile phone Sharmilla had given me and was managing to make and receive calls without a problem. This made communication between Trevor and I a lot easier and we could also call each other to say goodnight before we went off to sleep.

Trevor wanted to make sure Kristy would have access to a phone while she was in Richards Bay as well, so he put things in place to organise this for her. It would be much too expensive (as he'd found out firsthand) for her to use her Australian phone.

I hadn't seen Dr. Timakia or Dr. Lucelle for a few days and this was great because all was going so well. If the nurses had any concerns, they would have contacted them immediately.

On the Saturday morning, March 7, I awoke thinking how much more clarity of thought I had, and it hit me again how very lucky I was that I'd dodged a bullet.
I'd gotten up and had my usual morning bath. My roommate asked me a very simple question and suddenly I experienced a full-on setback. My mouth felt like it was filled with cotton wool. I knew what I wanted to say but couldn't bring the words forth. I clamped my mouth shut.

'Here I go again,' I thought.

I was frozen in fear! I had had such high hopes and couldn't believe this was starting to happen again. I told myself to stay calm, but I couldn't control the rush of negative thoughts that infiltrated my brain to the exclusion of any positive thoughts.

Hope left me, and in that instant, I was transported right back to the land of fear, doubt and uncertainty. I couldn't understand what had happened, and then just as quickly as it had come on, it left, and I could once again find my words and speak without any difficulty again as though nothing had happened. The whole incident lasted about 45 minutes.

I was scared to tell Dr. Timakia because if I told him, it would make it more real, and I didn't want it to be real. I wanted to be the 'miracle lady' and this would change that, I thought.

As it turned out, I didn't get to see him until the following morning and by that time I had a bit more to tell him.
Sunday morning, after a restless night, I got up, bathed and got dressed ready for this big day out. Going to church would be a wonderful way to start it. After yesterday's setback, I realised how quickly I could be enticed back into the land of fear and doubt, a land I'd lived in for far too long.

Dr. Lucelle had been called in to work, so we went to church with her husband, Kenneth.

Pastor Cecil Pillay was there to greet us as he did with his entire congregation. Music was playing. The singers were singing, and the vibe was there as it had been the week before. It was hard not to feel uplifted by the music, lights and atmosphere.

And then, I started to feel something coming over me. The lights flashing triggered something in my brain and the music and Pastor Cecil's voice started to become a faint sound in the distance as I slumped against Trevor's shoulder. My last words to him before I fainted were: 'I don't feel well.'

He was immediately alarmed as he watched me have a seizure. Fortunately, we were sitting in the back row and I only lost consciousness for about a minute, but it was enough to scare the life out of him.

None of the congregation saw what happened but Pastor Cecil acknowledged us and nodded his blessing as we quietly left the church.

We drove straight back to the hospital and Trevor spoke to the nursing staff and told them what had happened. They immediately contacted Dr. Timakia and he ordered a CT brain scan as well as several other tests just to make sure everything was healing okay and that I hadn't had a bleed or something untoward that had caused this.

The brain scan was very quick – no big clunky, noisy machines as before. It was just like having a photo taken (well maybe a bit more than that, but it was certainly no big deal). It showed that everything was healing well and there was no need for concern.

Trevor insisted I stay at the hospital and rest, and although I was disappointed I'd miss seeing him at Porky's (The Golf Club), I understood and didn't argue the point.

Obviously, his show was a great hit. As he always says: 'If you love what you're doing, it shows.'

Within an hour of me having my tests, Dr. Timakia came to see me and increased my dose of Epilim from 500mg to 700mg in the evening, keeping the morning dose at 500mg.

We discussed my seizure and I also decided to let good sense take over from fear and I told him about the incident a few days prior when I hadn't been able to find words or express myself verbally. He asked me how long it had lasted and whether I was aware of everything at the time. This apparently was a type of absence seizure. Although I was more concerned about the grand mal seizure I'd had the day before, he said this absent seizure was the one that concerned him more, but even that was to be expected because my brain was still very much at the beginning of the healing process.

He went on to explain that there were lots of different types of seizures (so many more than, even with my education, I was aware of). Anyway, the main thing now was to ensure my Epilim levels would be within therapeutic range so I would not have another seizure.

He said he was really pleased with my progress and that the seizure was something he expected. There was a huge space in my brain where the tumour had been and with the brain expanding to slowly fill up this space, it was not an unusual occurrence.

Having now had a seizure though, I was definitely not going to be able to drive for six months. If I had any more seizures, the six months would start from the date of the last one. For some reason, I believed that this would be a one-off incident.

There had been some articles we'd read recently about companion dogs and we told Dr. Timakia about our dog, Connie. She had developed this strange behavior of jumping up on my lap and sniffing at my head in a really insistent manner. It was strange enough for us to comment on it a number of times but all we did was wonder why she did it. It wasn't until all this had happened, we realised she was smarter than all of us. She knew something was seriously wrong way before any of us did.

He agreed there was certainly a lot of evidence supporting the value of dogs in diagnosing medical problems and assisting people by detecting when they were about to have a seizure. We thought we would do some more research and maybe our whippet girl, Connie would get herself a name as my companion dog.

Trevor continued writing his emails to people to keep them in the loop and it was great that he could now give them such good news. He knew that I still had a bit of a battle ahead of me physically, but each time he saw the spark in my eyes, it reminded him of the preciousness of life and not to ever take it, or our relationship, for granted. It was so wonderful that we had both been given this second chance.

A little over two weeks after my surgery, Dr. Timakia took out the rest of the staples and clips. There were a few stitches that needed removing, but he wanted to wait a little longer to take these out.

On the surface, everything was healing beautifully. There was no infection and he assured me he'd done his best to make sure the scar was not going to be visible after my hair grew again.

He showed Trevor and me the latest scans and we could see for ourselves that the midline was almost back to where it should be, smack bang in the middle of my brain, dividing the left and right hemispheres, rather than being pushed right over to one side.

While we were there, Trevor talked about how scary it was for him to see me have my seizure the day before. I had seen lots of people have various types of epileptic fits and it didn't frighten me, but I could understand where he was coming from. I tried to explain to him that just because this happened, he couldn't wrap me in cotton wool just in case it happened again.

I had a strange feeling just before hand and I knew that this was a good sign. This is known as an aura. Experiencing this means there is a bit of a warning just prior to a seizure.

I was completely on board with not driving and thought it would be totally irresponsible to drive when the risk of another seizure was so high. I would never have been able to forgive myself if I hurt or killed someone on the road just because of my stupidity.

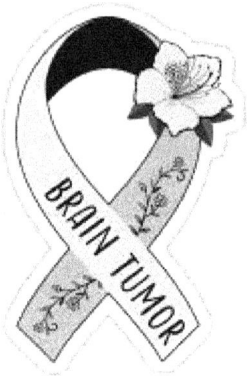

The world as you know it is

But a mere speck

In the realm of creativity;

Your life is but a speck of stardust,

But nonetheless paramount

In the purpose of things.

Remember to be in the instant only.

All that is past and all that is before you

Will unfold as it must.

Rely on the knowledge

That lies inert within you.

CHAPTER 21

The world will never be the same again

We started hearing lots more about coronavirus and it seemed there was more to this than any of us originally had thought. It wasn't just a nasty flu-type bug. It was something that seemed to be spreading like wildfire and it was becoming increasingly difficult to contain and control.

Initially we heard it had originated in Wuhan, China in December 2019, and in a statement, the World Health Organisation director-general Dr. Tedros Adhanom Ghebreyesus said: 'WHO has been assessing this outbreak around the clock and we are deeply concerned both by the alarming levels of spread and severity and by the alarming levels of inaction.'

By March 11, 2020 it had spread to more than 126,140 people across nearly 114 countries causing more than 4,600 deaths and as a result, WHO declared COVID-19 a global pandemic.

Things started to change in the hospital. Anyone entering the hospital had to register prior to entering and could only come in if they had a legitimate reason.

Visiting hours started to be limited as well and hand hygiene became compulsory as a condition of entry. Everyone had to have their temperatures taken prior to entry and anyone with a high temperature or symptoms had to be screened and tested for COVID-19.

Fortunately, Trevor was still able to have his usual long visits with me. Again, we were so grateful for these privileges we were given.

We had never witnessed anything like this, but even at this stage, we weren't aware of how much more serious it would become and how quickly this would happen.

Trevor was in constant contact with his Australian Princess cruising agent, Grayboy. They kept him updated and each time he called, things seemed to have changed. Cruise ships were not being allowed access into any of the ports, and the latest port to deny entry was The Seychelles, the next port of call where they were hoping he could embark.

Princess Cruises were busy looking at any and all alternatives but there were none. Trevor was more than happy to come on board to fulfil his contract, but this was literally impossible. It must have been a logistical nightmare for all concerned. The passengers who are used to a variety of entertainment would have nothing new for the rest of their trip and the entertainers who were on board would have to stay on board because there was nowhere to get off

In the meantime, Kristy was on her way over to Richards Bay and would be arriving on that same Wednesday, the Wednesday that COVID-19 was declared a pandemic. We were still oblivious to all the facts and were still living in our safe, secure, COVID-19-free bubble, oblivious to what lay in store.

I was so excited that I would be seeing Kristy. Secretly, I was glad Trevor was going to be there as well. She would have someone to look after her and it would not be as daunting an experience for her.

Although she had travelled by plane throughout Australia, her only overseas travel had been to Bali, a quick hop, skip and a jump from Townsville. She had done this accompanied by her partner, Mark, who was a very experienced traveller.

This would be her first ever experience travelling alone, halfway across the world to a country so similar, but also so different from Australia.

There was so much for her to sort out before she left. After all, she had four children, as well as a demanding cleaning business.

Initially she wasn't sure how long she'd be staying. All she knew was that I was definitely on the mend and she would be leaving the same time as me. Basically, it was dependent on Dr. Timakia giving the okay for me to fly home as well as a nurse being available to accompany me. It was still unclear whether Kristy would come home with me to the farm or whether, if Trevor wasn't able to do the next cruise (which seemed likely), he would accompany me, and she would fly straight home. We figured we would just wait and see.

Flying over was not the exciting adventure those who've never travelled imagine. It's so tiring, sitting cramped in economy class seating for hours on end. There were two legs to her journey and even though she was tired, her stopover in Dubai was one she did enjoy. Flying into Dubai was a unique experience and one she'd never forget. From the air, the sand dunes seemed to just go on and on. She had never seen anything like it. Then as she flew into Dubai Airport, she was surprised at the buildings that seemed to spring up out of nowhere. This city oozed prosperity.

The airport itself was unlike anything she'd seen in her life before. There were trains that went from one section of the airport to another, and she was so glad she had a bit of time up her sleeve so she could figure out where she had to be to get her next flight to Durban, where she'd be picked up by a port agent and taken to the lodge. She also had a chance to do a bit of duty-free shopping, something Dubai Airport is famous for.

I was so proud of her. She did all this like a seasoned traveller.

While she was on this arduous journey, Trevor and I were on a bit of an adventure as well. Pastor Cecil offered to take us on a safari.

We'd gone on a cruise around South Africa the year before and had booked a safari that we'd been really looking forward to. However, due to the fact that Princess Cruises weren't able to get any entertainers with a Brazilian visa and because we both have such a huge repertoire of material and still had a number of shows and talks up our sleeves, we'd been asked if we would extend our cruise an extra two weeks and go onto Brazil. They were obviously very grateful that we were happy to do this, as were the passengers.

There was no way we were going to give up that rare opportunity and the highlight for us would be seeing Saint Helena, a place rarely visited by tourists.

So, this time, although the circumstances were entirely different, we snapped up the opportunity to go on safari. It was such a kind and thoughtful gesture on behalf of Pastor Cecil.

We got to know him so much better as we drove out of town through some of the poorer parts of the area to Hluhluwei Mfolozi National Park, the oldest game reserve in Africa. We took heaps of photos and enjoyed every minute of the day we shared.

Despite not seeing any of the big five – elephant, lion, leopard, rhinoceros or buffalo – we saw lots of wildlife and just fell in love with the landscape, trees and foliage that make up the unique countryside that is South Africa.

Over a hearty late breakfast, we were captivated by Pastor Cecil's sensitivity and grasp of the human psyche. He seemed to have real insights into human suffering and frailties, and he projected an unconditional understanding. He understood all too well how the human soul becomes broken with rejection, depression and substance abuse. It was so uplifting and inspiring to be in his presence and we both loved his delightful sense of humour.

Although Kristy arrived on the Wednesday, she arrived in the evening, so I didn't get to see her until the following day. She rang me as soon as she arrived at the Indaba Lodge. I cried tears of joy, knowing she was safe and was finally here. Her voice was balm to my ears. I couldn't wait to see her.

Because Kristy had had such a long flight, she would likely be jetlagged so the plan was that she would have a sleep-in, followed by a leisurely breakfast with Trevor and then they would both come to see me the following day.

When she turned the corner to my room, my heart swelled with pride and love for her. I still couldn't believe she was finally here with me. I had bathed and had put on civvies that morning because I wanted her to see me up and about looking as healthy as I could. She immediately approved of my new hairstyle. She gave me a few hats and scarves she'd bought through the cancer online stores. They were fabulous. I was able to mix and match so I could look really chic, no matter what outfit I was wearing. I didn't know which one to wear first and I particularly loved a black and white one. It was thicker than the other two and it had the added advantage of cushioning and protecting my head at the same time. I got so many compliments when I wore them.

I knew that Dr. Timakia was coming in to see me and I was very keen for him to finally meet my girl. At the same time, he wanted me to meet his wife, Maya as well. Yes, amazingly, his wife had the same name as me (another extraordinary coincidence).

He'd obviously told her about 'this woman from Australia' who had caused him so many sleepless nights, and I figured she just wanted to see for herself the cause of his angst.

She was heavily pregnant and her beautiful baby boy was due to be born the following month. When she arrived, I could see what he saw in her. She was beautiful and it was obvious this beauty wasn't just skin-deep. Dr. Timakia stayed with us for a short time and then continued his rounds while she stayed behind and we all talked for what seemed like ages. Maya was just lovely and we really connected.

Initially he may have been a bit concerned about bringing her in to meet me, and he wanted to be sure we had no reservations about meeting her. After he explained her reason behind wanting to meet us, we were more than happy to oblige. In fact, we really wanted to do this. He said she had a friend who was a local journalist who wanted to write a newspaper article about us.

'Anything for a bit of attention,' I thought, and we certainly didn't mind a bit more attention being paid to us. After all, we were starting to get quite used to it! In all seriousness though, we were so grateful to everyone in this wonderful town with its people who had so generously opened their hearts up to us and had been part of our recent journey. We just wanted to tell anyone and everyone about our fabulous experience.

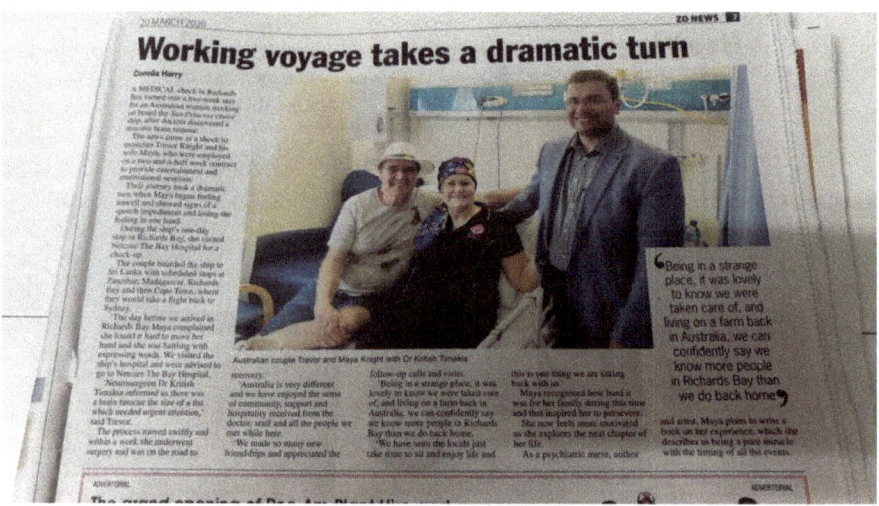

It was hard to believe we'd been in this place a month. We were so far from home, from family and friends and we had both changed and grown so much.

With COVID-19 looming as an unknown threat to the future of the world, we were unsure how we would be affected by it.

We still believed it would all go away as quickly as it had come, but it had other plans.

The cruising industry, which had been such a huge part of our lives and our financial security, was coming to a complete standstill, with passengers on board any of the ships that were sailing at the time, not knowing where or when they would be disembarking.

We really felt for those who had to try to manage this crisis, because not only did they have to keep paying passengers happy, they also had to accommodate a lot of passengers who were unable to fly (due to medical reasons) and continue to update and reassure future passengers as to what was going to happen (when they didn't have a clue themselves). The goalposts seemed to shift constantly.

It was now a definite that Trevor would be flying home with me, so we started to be more proactive with our plan to return home. Even though it would only end up a short stay, Kristy was going to fly back home to Townsville the following Monday, alone, not even five days after her arrival.

She contacted her travel agent as well as my insurance company and she then changed and confirmed her new departure date. Princess Cruises would again organise transport to Durban Airport for her and she would once again have to do the long journey back home. She would hardly have had time to get over jetlag, most might think. However, my girl is pretty tough and, just like us, she didn't seem to suffer it – a real blessing.

We didn't want to waste any of the time while she was there, and although she had other ideas, I wanted for her to see this as a holiday. She kept saying she was there for me and just wanted to spend the time with me.

We went to the mall most days, had lunch at *The Elephant and I* and we introduced her to our newfound friends. Trevor showed her some of the sights in the vicinity of the lodge and the two of them went for long walks in the evening after they returned there.

Outside the lodge, swinging from tree to tree were a family of monkeys. This was quite a common sight and although tempted, they did not engage or feed them. The monkeys would play hide and seek, and they said it was so funny watching the juvenile monkeys up to their cute little tricks.

Kristy was a real hit with Sharmilla and Angelique and they were keen to take her out. They arranged to treat her to a day out at Emdoneni Wildcat Project, a small sanctuary where she would have the opportunity to see cheetahs, lynx and other African wildcats. When she told me where they wanted to take her, she was so excited. This had always been on her wish list and now she would be able to tick it off. When she told her boys, they were so envious and made her promise to take lots of photos.

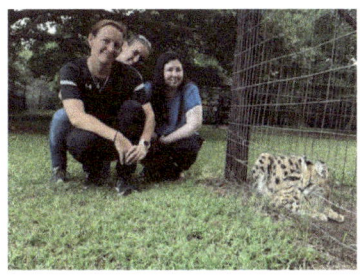

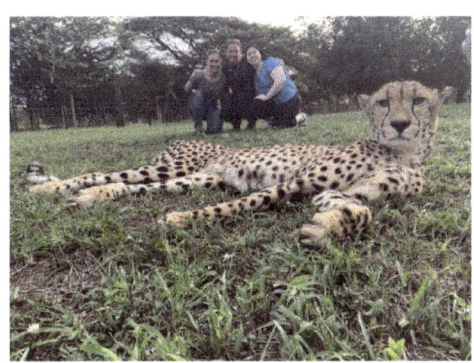

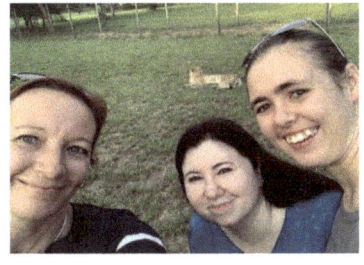

She had the most amazing time. When she returned, she could hardly stop talking about it. She had been so surprised at how close they'd been allowed to get to these wild animals. Although they had to be aware at all times and weren't allowed to stroke some of the big cats, she said it was amazing when some of the big kitties gently rubbed up against her.

She loved being with both Sharmilla and Angelique and could understand why Trevor and I thought so highly of them – they were (and are) very special indeed.

I had to laugh when she told me they had tried to introduce her to the local alcohol which, not wanting to be impolite, she had to accept.

Each day with her was special. If I thought we were close before, I realised that now we were even closer. This whole experience had done this for us. Not only this, but it had also brought her and Trevor closer. He got to know her and see her in a new light.

She is and always has been my shining light and it was so great that others had the opportunity to see her as I always have.

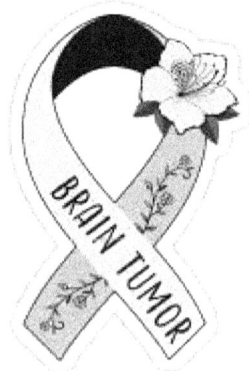

You will suffer with the fall and be strengthened
By the growth and promise of spring
For everything there is a time
And morning comes after each passing day

All that is needed is a firm belief
That whatever the Universe
Determines your fate to be

Is exactly what you need to embrace,

With light, truth, hope and love.

CHAPTER 22

It's now or never

Saying goodbye to Kristy was bittersweet. I was so glad she'd come over to see me and I knew this was a real milestone in our relationship. I knew how much she'd sacrificed to do this, and knowing this, made me appreciate her and what she'd done even more.

She'd put her life on hold and had faced her fear of travelling halfway across the world on her own. She's such an inspiration to me.

On the Monday morning, she packed her bags and came to visit me at the hospital for the last time. Trevor and I were planning to leave on Wednesday, March 18 and hopefully a nurse would have been arranged to fly with me by that time. Dr. Timakia was working on it in conjunction with the insurance company, but nothing had been put in place that we knew of at this stage.

When Kristy walked in that last day, I was reminded of my excitement at seeing her just a few days prior to this, and again I marvelled at how much could change so quickly.

I was also aware that it wasn't likely I would see her for some time. After all, we live 2,000 kilometres from each other, and both have commitments that keep us at home. I was happy for her though, knowing she would soon see her children and partner again, and that life for her would get back to normal. I knew she'd missed her family and she was keen to take up where she'd left off.

We had a final lunch and then she was picked up from the hospital and her arduous journey home commenced.

By the time Kristy had gotten to Dubai Airport we all knew she would have to be in quarantine for two weeks. She wouldn't be able to be in close contact with her family for a fortnight. Those hello hugs and wonderful-to-have-you-home cuddles would have to wait.

Fortunately, Mark, her partner was onto it and although not what he wanted, she was able to stay at his mother's house for the compulsory two-week period. She wasn't able to even go to the grocery store and work was out of the question. I felt so guilty about this, but she reassured me that even if she'd known this would have been the outcome, she would still have gone. For her there was no doubt at all as to where she belonged and when I needed her most, she was there with, and for me.

That afternoon, we wanted to say our goodbyes to all the nurses who, in our eyes, had been God-sent. We went to the emergency department first and although I couldn't remember some of the nurses' names, they remembered us with fond memories and wished us all the very best. It was hard to believe as we walked back into this section of the hospital, that the last time I had been here, I'd come in on a stretcher, not knowing what was wrong with me and with no idea of what was ahead of me. I had been on an amazing journey in my heart, body and soul. This whole experience had such a huge impact on me, and I know it did as well on all those close to me, for the better.

My next port of call was the ICU. This had been my safe haven. This was where I faced my darkest fears and looked them straight in the eye. This was where I had comforting hands that soothed me, bathed me, dressed me and supported me when I couldn't do this for myself. This was where I was constantly monitored and had my every need attended to. This was where I left a big part of my heart. Without the staff from ICU, I wouldn't be alive to tell this tale. They took care of all the day-to-day things and they encouraged me to do more and be more every day. They gave me my second chance at life, and every day I live, I remember this and give thanks.

Unfortunately, when I got there, there were only a handful of the nurses I'd grown to know and love. I was so sad not to be able to say a personal thank you and goodbye to everyone, but I know in the nursing game, people are on other shifts or have days off.

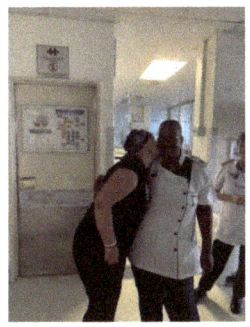

After this we went to the hospital pharmacy and collected all of my discharge medication.

Then we went to the hospital cafeteria for a wonderful cup of coffee and a piece of their special carrot cake. This cake is so yummy – it's almost worth being in hospital or visiting the hospital for. After saying goodbye and thank you to them as well, I went back to the ward and Trevor went back to the lodge.

The situation with COVID-19 was hotting up even more and we knew by that afternoon that we had to move quickly to get ourselves out of the country. It was getting critical, and we were hearing things that gravely concerned us.

I stayed in hospital that night and Trevor notified the insurance company about his concerns. They were quite blasé about the situation. They said they had things in hand and were organising a nurse to be flown out from Canada to Richards Bay where she or he would stay overnight and assess me and then fly home with me on the Friday.

They just didn't seem to understand that it might be too late if we went by their schedule.

The next day we knew without a doubt that we couldn't wait any longer – if we did, who knew when we would be able to get home?

Trevor got on the phone to Cover-More yet again only this time with much more urgency in his tone and demeanour. He told me that he had tried to rationalise with them and get them to understand our very real predicament and the urgency of the situation, but they just weren't hearing him. He even phoned Dr. Timakia and got him to phone them as well and they weren't hearing him either.

Because the internet and phone coverage at Indaba Lodge was better than at the hospital, Trevor stayed there all day trying to sort it out. Even so, phone calls cut out from time to time as well, adding to his frustration.

I remained at the hospital while all this was happening, once again not totally aware of the severity of things or the way things were escalating.

Later that day, Dr. Timakia came into the hospital to see me and on Trevor's request, he made a point of amending the forms so rather than stating that I needed a nurse to accompany me home, it now read that I could fly unaccompanied as long as I was in business class and Trevor was with me.

This was emailed to the insurance company and even then, the insurance company was reluctant. In fact, they paid it no heed, insisting they'd been in contact with the Australian government, and all would be fine for me to fly home later that week as per their initial arrangement.

On the one hand we understood that they needed to follow procedure and normal protocol, but this was a situation unlike any other. If we didn't go soon, who knew what could happen?

By Tuesday morning, we knew without a doubt that the airport was closing on the Wednesday, and when Trevor told them this, they wouldn't believe it.

They assured Trevor it wouldn't be a problem, to which Trevor replied: 'But you're not here and we know for a fact there will be no flights home after tomorrow.'

They just stuck to their guns and said: 'Well that's what's going to happen! You have to wait for the nurse to come from Canada and he or she will escort Maya on the plane as per our previous conversation.'

Can you imagine Trevor's frustration?

He didn't know how he was going to get through to them, but he knew he had to, one way or another.

He was losing charge on his phone and his credits were running out rapidly.

He asked the insurance company to phone him back and there were huge delays in them getting back to him.

In the meantime, he also heard that the Indaba Lodge would be closing down and the drivers were very concerned that they would lose their jobs.

I phoned Trevor at one stage to see what was happening and he nearly bit my head off as he told me in no uncertain terms he couldn't talk at that time. He had to get things sorted with the insurance company and they just weren't listening.

He was waiting for yet another call from them, and this went on for hours.

In the end, Dr. Timakia once again became our saviour. He told them he had not only amended the form to read I could now fly unassisted; he had signed it as well and he (with the agreement of myself and Trevor) would take all responsibility should anything untoward happen to me. This would mean the insurance company was not liable. He was pretty insistent, if you get my drift...

Finally, just after 4pm, after hours of negotiating, they finally relented – and not a moment too soon.

Trevor had been aware all along of the dire consequences to us if we hadn't been allowed to leave – no home (Indaba Lodge would be closed), no transport and no means of getting home to Australia while living in a country where COVID-19 was starting to rear its ugly head. The ramifications were unthinkable.

Dr. Timakia officially discharged me, and I organised transport to the Indaba Lodge where Trevor was waiting for me.

As I walked out of the hospital doors, the first case of COVID-19 walked in.

What were the chances? I marvelled again at my luck; or was it divine intervention or simply the Universe taking care of us?

I gave thanks once again for all these coincidences.

When I arrived at Indaba Lodge, Trevor and I took some time to just be there for each other and although we knew we weren't home and hosed yet, we knew we were on our way. I was so proud of Trevor. He was my constant throughout this whole ordeal and never once waivered in his resolve to be his best and give of his best always. I truly understood the term unconditional love, because I had been the recipient of it.

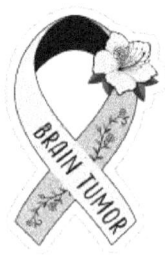

A calendar is only a reminder of the passage

of time

Everything happens exactly as it should

And your hand does little

To forward the hands of time.

This in itself is useful in that you can be open to

change

Knowing in your heart that significant events

Will indeed befall you and will have an impact

On your being

CHAPTER 23

Up, up and away

The insurance company were fabulous in emailing the details of our flights and, because our first flight left at 8.50am from Durban, which is at least a 2.5-hour drive away and we were **not** going to miss it, we decided to set the alarm for 2.30am. This would give us time to get ready and we would have plenty of time up our sleeves should anything go wrong on the way. Our driver had agreed to come and collect us at 3am.

We had already packed everything, so all we needed to do was put some personal, last-minute items in the suitcase and do what we always call an 'idiot check', just to make sure nothing had been left behind.

So much had transpired that day. Trevor was mentally exhausted. He fell into a fitful sleep and when he finally managed to get to sleep, the loud ringing of the phone woke him from his deep slumber. He was expecting the gentle, soft and gradual waking of the alarm but instead he woke up with a real start.

The voice on the phone was a female, Australian voice. She said: 'I'm ringing to inform you that the flight from Durban to Johannesburg you were booked on at 8.50am has been cancelled. The only flight that is available is at 6am. If you miss this, there will be no more flights."

He looked at the clock. It was midnight.

This would give us four hours to get ready, phone the driver, have him come from the other side of town, pick us up and then drive us to Durban Airport.

We didn't have a moment to waste.

Just when we thought nothing else could possibly go wrong, it did. Here we were, faced with yet another huge setback.

As Trevor phoned the driver, we prayed as never before, that he would answer.

We didn't know what we would do if he didn't.

Once again, there was someone looking after us.

The poor driver had hardly had any sleep himself and, understanding the urgency of our situation, and hearing the desperation in Trevor's voice, he rushed over as quickly as he could. We were amazed just how quickly he had gotten there and didn't dare ask if he'd violated any speeding limits. All we knew was that he was there, and he'd arrived safely to take us where we needed to go.

When he arrived, he helped us put the luggage in the car and seeing we were safely in the car, the driver immediately put the car in gear and we were off, roaring through the night along the freeway towards Durban Airport and the last plane that was there waiting for us.

His eyes were bloodshot from lack of sleep and we knew it must have taken every ounce of intestinal fortitude to stay awake.

I sat in the front and I lay the chair back so that I could get more comfortable. It was still difficult to get my head in a position that didn't hurt because it remained extremely tender along my suture line and also where the drains had been. I tried to avoid the hard surfaces on the edges of the car seat and I also found these tender areas of my head were consistently being knocked against the window as well. It's a bit like when you stub your toe and that's what you'll knock over and over again.

I couldn't believe it when the thought crossed my mind that I really missed my hospital bed and pillows. It was only a temporary thought though, and I soon replaced it with the fantasy and realisation that within the next few days, I would be home again in my own bed, with my own pillows, with the love of my life, Trevor lying beside me. That was such a comforting thought.

As our driver pulled up at Durban Airport, we checked our watches. We were running out of time and had to rush to get to the gate.

We heard the announcement then over the loudspeaker: 'Would Mr Trevor Knight and Mrs Maya Knight please go to the check-in counter as your flight is about to close.'

We got there by the skin of our teeth.

Trevor knew I would need help getting to and onto the plane because I was still quite weak. The lack of sleep hadn't helped matters much either. He arranged for an attendant to come with a wheelchair and assist me, while he followed, carrying our onboard luggage.

The flight to Johannesburg was short and uneventful. This filled me with confidence, knowing I'd been in the air without a hint of a seizure. Two more flights and we would be touching down in Sydney – and then only a short 250-kilometre drive home via ambulance.

We swore we would kiss the ground when we arrived home.

After our initial rush of getting to Durban Airport and finally getting all our luggage tagged and booked to go all the way through to Sydney, what we were met with in Johannesburg, was a completely different scenario and certainly not what we expected.

Because of our early arrival from Durban and the scheduled flight from Johannesburg being the same, we had to wait for about two hours before they even opened the check-in counter.

We thought we'd hit a ghost town. What would normally be a bustling hive of commuters was now a trickle of diehard travellers.

There was a real sense of impending doom. It was almost like the last day.

There were people desperately trying to get home and needing to get flights out of South Africa.

At last, it was time to board our plane, a beautiful Singapore Airways Silverbird, an 8380 Airbus.

As we walked through the entrance to business class seating, we felt so welcomed and spoilt by each of the flight attendants who looked after us. Nothing was too much trouble as they enveloped us in the lap of luxury in this dome of safety, peace and tranquility on board the airbuses that would be taking us home.

It was interesting to note we had arrived in Richards Bay on February 17 and here we were leaving on March 17, exactly one calendar month later.

It was almost surreal when we looked back and realised that, in reality, getting the very last flight home at the outbreak of COVID-19 had indeed been a mission almost impossible … Tom Cruise, eat your heart out.

We had gone through so much and all with the support and love of our friends and family as well as the special people of this wonderful rainbow nation. We'd grown to love them all and knew they would forever hold a special place in our hearts.

Over the years, we have visited many places throughout the world, but we have **never** met such wonderful and friendly folks as we did in Richards Bay. They opened their hearts to us and as a result we have made lifelong friends.

Wow! What an incredible journey this had been, from the depths of despair to the heights of new beginnings and hope for what lies ahead.

We learned the true meaning of unconditional love, to never take anything for granted and to face your fears full-on with courage, faith and hope.

Our departure was bittersweet, for as we were heading east into the rising sun, below us, who knew what was happening to our friends as the dark cloud of COVID-19 rolled over South Africa?

THE END

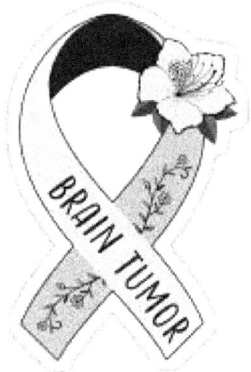

THE AFTERMATH

Arriving back in Australia was like coming into a world we hardly knew – one where rationing had become a reality, with toilet paper and rice in great demand and very difficult to come by.

We could never have envisaged such dramatic changes could have become a reality for so many people – some for the better and some certainly for the worse.

Trevor and I started to really appreciate all the smaller things. Where we were once caught up in a rat race of our own making, we now found ourselves valuing each other more and finding joy in the simpler things life had to offer.

I had come through such a special experience and the way I described this was that there was now a fragility that existed for me.

The experience had shown me that we are each very fragile in our own way. We never know when disaster might strike and when we might lose something very dear to us.

It showed me how fragile relationships are and how much we rely on love of family and friends. I understood their value in supporting me and giving me strength. They helped me overcome adversity and gave me something to look forward to.

I also found that I had a strength within me that seemed to know no bounds and these compensated for any physical strength that left me in the initial stages.

Hans and Rowena were with us for the first few months of my recovery and were an absolute God send for us. I think that when they'd first heard of my diagnosis, and after seeing the rapid progression of my symptoms, they were not very optimistic with regard to me making such a quick and steady recovery and they continued to be surprised as they witnessed it first hand.

We were so grateful to them for dropping everything and being with us for the first 2 months after we came home. They were such a wonderful support to both of us, and our lives were all the richer for that very special time we shared together.

After selling their house in Brisbane they took up a bit of a nomadic life travelling the East coast of Australia as they waited for their new home to be built.

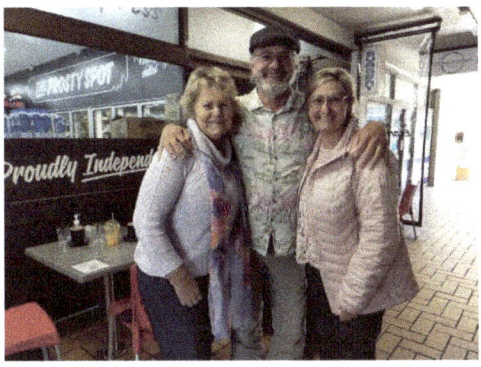

Hans and Rowena once we were home.

When we compared ourselves with the rest of the world, we realised again that we live in the *Lucky Country*. We have such amazing open spaces and a culture of people who, for the most part, are happy to comply with measures taken by the Government to prevent cross infection. We have a very stable economy and during the worst of it, businesses and individuals were supported through a very generous social security system.

I was unable to work for at least 6 months and who knew what was going to happen for Trevor. He had worked in the cruising industry as well as the entertainment industry and both of these were now defunct.

Travel overseas was very restricted and then stopped. Even travel within the country across state borders required a legitimate reason and permit and borders between states were continually closing at a few hours notice to contain this deadly virus.

We had to look at other options. Without a regular income and no Fairy Godmother, we had no money coming in. Hans, having a background in social work, tackled the mountain of paperwork and jumped through the many hoops it took for us to become eligible for any benefits. We then had to wait another few weeks for money to come through.

Although much less than what we were used to, we were grateful none-the-less. We thought of the other countries throughout the world more seriously affected by this pandemic with people not having ready access to Government funds the way we did.

Having developed a very good reputation over the years as a nurse, I had no problem being reinstated and before the year was up, I was back to working on a casual basis doing almost full-time hours.

I could say it was all plain sailing and that there were absolutely no repercussions but that would be sugar-coating things. After all, I'd had a huge part of my skull actually cut out and removed as well as a tumour the size of a tennis ball taken out. Naturally it would take time for my skull to fuse together and my brain to readjust so it would sit normally within my skull.

Some of my issues at the beginning were:
- I sometimes had periods of insomnia
- My right hand would often become numb followed by the most excruciating pain in my hand.
- Sometimes I got things mixed up. Eg. When I tried to open our gate at home (despite having done it thousands of times) I would go to the opposite side.
- I had some difficulty with depth perception –stepping down from any height can still be quite difficult for me.
- I had bouts of dizziness.
- Although not having any headaches or pain, my head still remains tender and I have had to change my sleeping position to avoid any discomfort or pain.
- From time to time, I forgot how to do things that were second nature to me, so I have had to re-learn them.

These issues were minor to me though, because ultimately I could manage every one of them. They were such a small price to pay for my life.

As my tomorrows became todays and my todays became yesterdays, 2 days really stood out for me.

The first was when I went to my hairdresser, Cheryl for the first time after having had all my hair shaved off.

She showed me such compassion and as she shampooed my short, now very curly hair and cut it into a cute pixie style, I felt a bond of trust grow between us.

She was so gentle and understanding and this was something I appreciated so much at this time. I felt tears well in my eyes sitting in her hairdressing chair remembering the last time I'd sat there all those months ago.

So much had happened since then and it was like my hair, the loss of it and its ability to grow back strong and resilient were all so symbolic of the changes that had also occurred within me.

The second very significant day was when I had my first MRI brain scan in Australia, 6 months after my surgery. I knew what to expect having had two in South Africa, so I certainly wasn't expecting this rush of emotions that came over me suddenly and totally without warning.

I couldn't understand nor make sense of my feelings. It was like I was right back where I'd started with all the fears of not knowing what the results would be. I felt so fragile.

I knew in my head that I'd overcome so much and that I was well on the mend.

However, it was like the month I'd been in Richards Bay had compressed itself together as I lay inside the MRI machine that clanged and clunked around me, oblivious to my internal conflict and distress.

As I was taken out of the machine, I could hold it back no longer and I felt the tears of sadness and relief, fear and gratitude roll down my cheeks. It was such a cathartic experience and obviously one I needed to tie everything neatly together for me.

Over time, I have been able to stay in touch with most of the people who'd touched our lives so profoundly.

Dr. Timakia continues to work tirelessly and is now the proud father a little boy, Sharaav born 9th April 2020.

Angelique is still a paramedic and continues to witness so much more in her day-to-day job, especially with cases and different strains of Covid-19 being on the rise.

Sharmila and I have maintained regular contact and I was really sad to hear that she'd been diagnosed positive of Covid-

19 and her recovery took several months in which time she was very sick. Even now she is still not her full, vibrant self – something a lot of people who've been diagnosed Covid-19 positive complain of.

Tristan continues to excel in his job as a Pathologist and has recently gained much recognition internationally for his contributions as a teacher. He and his wife Rene and their 3 children recently bought their own home so life is really going forward for them.

Kristy and I have seen each other a few times since our time in South Africa and we continue to have such a strong bond because of it. Her business is doing well and her children are all excelling at work, school as well as the various sports they do. The 3 youngest represent North Queensland in soccer and basketball.

Steven continues to live with Kristy and has got himself a great job and now drives a pretty flash Subaru.

Bronwyn continues to work as a Veterinary Specialist in Canada and although loving her work, she was quite concerned with the rising cases of Covid-19 and her inability to be vaccinated till months after the vaccination had been made available. She loves her life with her husband, Tony and their horses. The only thing that would make her happier is to once again be able to travel and spend that one-on-one time with her family and friends in Australia.

Trevor and I found even greater hidden depths to our talents. I took up painting again – something that I'd let slide in the few years prior to my diagnosis and I have also authored this book you hold in your hands.

We both realised the precious gift our property is to us and decided we would share its uniqueness for others to enjoy as well.

Although we bred our whippets and our horses on it, we realised there was so much more it had to offer. Nestled in the middle of a National Park surrounded on three sides by native trees, it truly is 'Our Little Piece of Heaven'.

We decided to join Hip-camp and now have groups of people who camp on our property and get a taste of what we enjoy every day. This really made us see and appreciate what we owned in a whole new light.

We have met so many interesting people through opening up our property to Hip-campers. Trevor has done his various shows on a more intimate level and has done Horse Whispering demonstrations to various groups as well. He continues to write and record more music and in my opinion, just like a fine whisky – he just keeps improving with age.

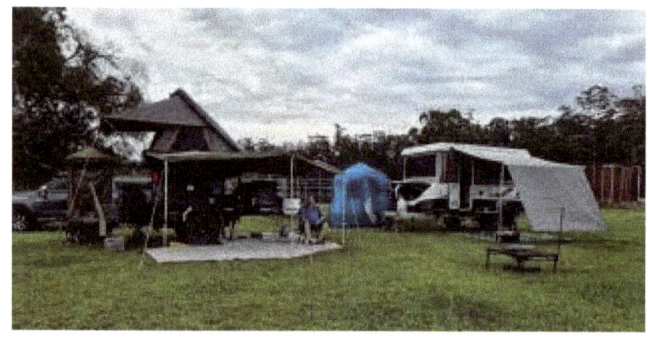

Hip-camp.

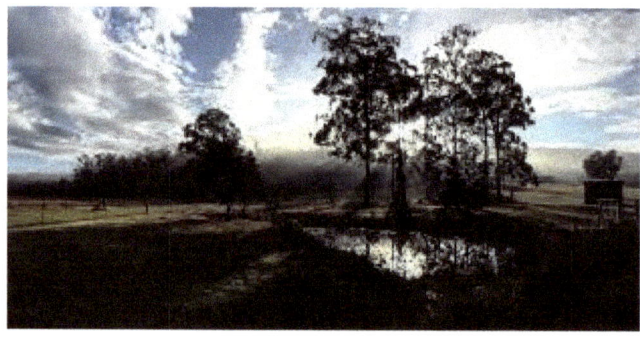

Life as we knew it on the high seas may be a thing of the past, but our memories are filled with the many experiences and people we met on our travels.

We are both firm believers that 'when one door closes, another one opens' and we both know we have so many doors and windows opening for both of us.

Each sunrise to us heralds the beginning of a new day and these days, each day is filled with promise of challenges, joys and new experiences.

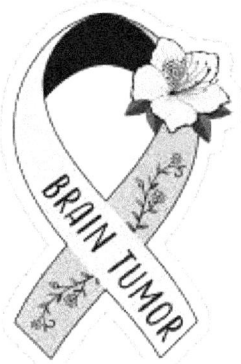

www.ingramcontent.com/pod-product-compliance
Lightning Source LLC
Chambersburg PA
CBHW051534010526
44107CB00064B/2723